AF905641

Updates in Surgery

The aim of this series is to provide informative updates on hot topics in the areas of breast, endocrine, and abdominal surgery, surgical oncology, and coloproctology, and on new surgical techniques such as robotic surgery, laparoscopy, and minimally invasive surgery. Readers will find detailed guidance on patient selection, performance of surgical procedures, and avoidance of complications. In addition, a range of other important aspects are covered, from the role of new imaging tools to the use of combined treatments and postoperative care.

The topics addressed by volumes in the series Updates in Surgery have been selected for their broad significance in collaboration with the Italian Society of Surgery. Each volume will assist surgical residents and fellows and practicing surgeons in reaching appropriate treatment decisions and achieving optimal outcomes. The series will also be highly relevant for surgical researchers.

Diego Cuccurullo • Corrado Rispoli
Editors

Complex Abdominal Wall Surgery

Springer

SOCIETÀ ITALIANA DI CHIRURGIA
FONDATA A ROMA NEL 1882

Editors
Diego Cuccurullo
Unit of General,
Laparoscopic and Robotic Surgery
A.O.R.N. dei Colli Monaldi Hospital
Naples, Italy

Corrado Rispoli
Unit of General,
Laparoscopic and Robotic Surgery
A.O.R.N. dei Colli Monaldi Hospital
Naples, Italy

ISSN 2280-9848 ISSN 2281-0854 (electronic)
Updates in Surgery
ISBN 978-3-032-24283-9 ISBN 978-3-032-24284-6 (eBook)
https://doi.org/10.1007/978-3-032-24284-6

This work was supported by Italian Society of Surgery.

The Editors of the volume and the Italian Society of Surgery would like to thank Assut Europe S.p.A., Becton Dickinson Italia S.p.A., Johnson & Johnson MedTech (a branch of Johnson and Johnson Medical S.p.A.) and Maya Pharma S.r.l. for their unconditional contribution, which made it possible to publish this book under the Open Access model.

This Springer imprint is published by the registered company Springer Nature Switzerland AG
The registered company address is: Gewerbestrasse 11, 6330 Cham, Switzerland

Foreword

It is with sincere satisfaction that I introduce this volume by Diego Cuccurullo and Corrado Rispoli, published on the occasion of the presentation of his Biennial Report at the 128th Congress of the Italian Society of Surgery, a forum for research, education, and clinical innovation in the surgical field.

This work brings together contributions from authors of proven expertise, each providing a qualified and highly specialized perspective on some of the most complex and challenging topics in modern surgery, abdominal wall reconstruction in its most advanced forms, which today represents a true discipline in its own right, owing to its scientific content, clinical criticalities, and impact on patients' quality of life.

Indeed, the objective is not merely the repair of an anatomical defect, but the restoration of a biomechanical, functional, and systemic equilibrium, often compromised by previous surgical interventions, infections, and other pathological conditions, including, among others, obesity and the sequelae of prior procedures, even involving prosthetic materials.

This volume is commendable for addressing these issues through a systemic, multidisciplinary, and evidence-based approach.

Following the essential foundations and core principles—indispensable cultural and methodological premises—the text proceeds to an introductory framework of complex abdominal wall surgery, outlining the classification criteria that guide appropriate clinical decision-making. Particular attention is given to biomechanical alterations and systemic effects, emphasizing that a parietal defect should not be considered an isolated event, but rather a condition capable of influencing respiration, posture, visceral dynamics, and the patient's overall functional performance.

Of particular contemporary relevance are preoperative planning and risk stratification, areas in which advanced imaging, functional assessment, and prognostic scoring systems constitute indispensable tools for tailoring therapeutic strategies. This section is complemented by an analysis of surgical anatomy, reinterpreted from a functional and reconstructive perspective, forming the essential foundation of any high-complexity procedure.

The volume rigorously addresses surgical strategies. From the open approach, with its various mesh placement options and advanced reconstructive techniques, the discussion extends to laparoscopic and robotic procedures, expressions of technological progress that have expanded therapeutic possibilities while reducing invasiveness.

Special emphasis is placed on the selection of prosthetic materials—biological, synthetic, and hybrid—a crucial aspect in the prevention of complications and the durability of outcomes.

The management of large incisional hernias and parastomal hernias is presented with a pragmatic and innovative approach, offering technical solutions tailored to highly complex clinical scenarios.

The most challenging situations are then examined: mesh infections, chronic complications related to prosthetic materials, enterocutaneous and abdominal fistulas, and surgery in obese or bariatric patients. These conditions require advanced, multidisciplinary expertise, as well as decision-making skills developed in high-volume, specialized settings.

The integrated approach proposed by the authors highlights how the management of these conditions must rely on structured care pathways, careful risk–benefit balancing, and rigorous patient selection.

Finally, the last section projects the discipline toward future perspectives. Tissue engineering and regenerative medicine open scenarios of extraordinary interest, in which stem cells, scaffolds, and advanced biomaterials may redefine the paradigms of abdominal wall reconstruction.

In parallel, the adoption of Enhanced Recovery After Surgery (ERAS) protocols in abdominal wall reconstruction underscores the importance of organizational innovation capable of improving clinical outcomes, reducing complications, and optimizing resource utilization.

This volume stands as the expression of a cohesive scientific community, sharing language, methodology, and objectives. The plurality of contributions converges into a unified vision: patient-centered care, methodological rigor, multidisciplinary integration, and a constant commitment to improving outcomes.

President of the Italian Society of Surgery Ludovico Docimo
Naples, Italy
September 2026

Foreword

It is a true pleasure and an honor to present this remarkable monograph, edited by my dear friend Professor Diego Cuccurullo and his associate Corrado Rispoli. This work provides an invaluable overview of all aspects of this significant and common pathological condition and its surgery.

Written in a clear and informative style, this work is timely and very useful, as it reflects the several rapid conceptual progressions, technical evolutions, and outcome improvements that this surgery has recently undergone. In the volume's precise and well-structured 4 parts and 15 chapters, the editors and prominent Italian and international authors, all leading experts in their field, deal with all aspects of complex abdominal wall defects and reconstructive procedures and answer the many questions that this topic poses. The result is a volume that is highly interesting to read and study.

Part I starts with a comprehensive introduction that defines the disease and explains its clinical significance, before going on to describe the surgical anatomy and pathophysiology, preoperative planning, and risk stratification.

Part II—perhaps the most captivating and engaging—looks at clinical strategies and surgical techniques. It provides a thorough overview of all open, laparoscopic, and robotic surgical techniques with a precise breakdown of the technical steps for each type of abdominal wall defect, as well as a detailed analysis of the indications, advantages, and disadvantages of all prosthetic materials currently used in our operating rooms.

Part III discusses in great detail particular scenarios and complications associated with this surgery, while Part IV closes the book by opening up to future prospects and innovative technologies, such as tissue engineering.

The authors are to be congratulated on the high quality of their work. I am sure this up-to-date and easy-to-read text will become a reference that will captivate readers, both non-expert and advanced ones alike.

I am also convinced that this book will be a milestone and will not suffer the same fate as some other similar works, for which *the sands of time were eroded by the river of constant change...*

President Emeritus of the Italian Society of Surgery — Massimo Carlini
Rome, Italy
September 2026

Foreword

It is both a great honor and a genuine pleasure to introduce this volume on Complex Abdominal Wall Surgery, entrusted to the expertise, vision, and dedication of my longstanding close collaborator, Diego Cuccurullo. Over the years, he has consistently stood at the forefront of progress in general surgery and, in particular, in abdominal wall surgery, contributing to the development and dissemination of innovations and technical refinements that, until relatively recently, would have seemed scarcely conceivable.

When I began my surgical career, abdominal wall surgery was regarded as a marginal field, attracting limited interest among surgeons and relying on a small number of conventional techniques that were frequently associated with unsatisfactory outcomes. The subsequent introduction of prosthetic materials, followed by minimally invasive approaches and, more recently, robotic surgery, has profoundly transformed this discipline. Today, abdominal wall surgery represents a major priority within the surgical community, owing to the increasing complexity of procedures and the technological sophistication required, establishing it as a highly specialized field reserved for dedicated experts.

I clearly recall that, during my training, complex incisional hernias were often considered unsuitable for surgical repair. Operative treatment was frequently discouraged because of technical challenges and the high risk of recurrence. Although these conditions remain demanding and, at times, difficult to manage, contemporary surgeons can now rely on advanced and refined techniques that enable complex abdominal wall reconstructions, restoring strength, functionality, and physiological compliance to the abdominal wall.

For many years, Diego Cuccurullo and his team have represented a recognized point of reference within the European landscape of abdominal wall surgery. I am therefore particularly gratified that this important responsibility has been entrusted to him and I wish to express my sincere appreciation to the Italian Society of Surgery for offering him this prestigious opportunity.

My warmest thanks and congratulations extend to the editors and, above all, to the authors who have contributed to this monograph, which fully reflects the scientific rigor and academic standards that characterize the Biennial Reports of the Italian Society of Surgery.

I am firmly convinced that this book will become a cornerstone in the education of surgeons and an essential reference for all those wishing to deepen their understanding of the complex and fascinating challenges of abdominal wall surgery.

Naples, Italy
September 2026

Francesco Corcione

Preface

Editing a volume dedicated to complex abdominal wall surgery represents not only a scientific challenge but also an acknowledgment of the clinical relevance that this field has progressively acquired within modern surgery.

For a long time, abdominal wall surgery was not recognized as a distinct field within general surgery. Opening and closing the abdomen were traditionally considered fundamental skills, part of the basic surgical armamentarium that every resident was expected to master at the very beginning of their training. The abdominal wall has often been perceived as a simple anatomical barrier rather than as a complex functional structure whose integrity is essential for respiration, movement, posture, and quality of life. As a result, defects of the abdominal wall were frequently approached with very few standardized, sometimes reductive solutions, with poor long-term functional and biological consequences.

This perception began to change with recognition of the abdominal wall as an organ and an increased understanding of its anatomy and function, thus, with the evolution of new technologies. Among these, robotic surgery has succeeded in overcoming the limitations of laparoscopy, allowing the reproduction of all procedural steps that could previously be performed only in open surgery.

At the same time, surgeons are now facing an increasingly complex and comorbid patient population, in which cardiovascular, respiratory, metabolic, and nutritional impairments are the rule rather than the exception, making a truly multidisciplinary approach mandatory. Furthermore, abdominal wall surgery has arguably become the field with the widest range of contemporary available techniques, often coexisting rather than replacing one another. This extraordinary technical diversity, while offering tailored solutions, also makes the discipline particularly demanding, as it can no longer be effectively practiced without a thorough knowledge of dozens of reconstructive strategies.

This volume reflects this evolution and aims to provide a structured framework for navigating the "uncharted" territory of complex abdominal wall surgery.

Naples, Italy — Diego Cuccurullo
Naples, Italy — Corrado Rispoli
September 2026

Contents

Part I

Fundamentals and Basic Principles

Introduction to Complex Abdominal Wall Surgery: Definition, Epidemiology, and Clinical Relevance

1

Diego Cuccurullo

1.1 Introduction

Complex abdominal wall (CAW) surgery has emerged over the last three decades as a distinct and increasingly important subspecialty within general surgery. Advances in surgical techniques, biomaterials, and perioperative care have significantly improved outcomes for patients with abdominal wall defects; nevertheless, the management of complex cases continues to represent a formidable challenge. The term "CAW surgery" refers not only to technical difficulties related to closure and reconstruction, but also to the multifactorial clinical scenarios in which these defects occur.

Patients with CAW conditions often present with multiple comorbidities, prior surgical history, chronic infection or enteric fistulas, making operative planning and execution extremely challenging. At the same time, the growing prevalence of obesity, the aging surgical population, and the increased survival of patients after major abdominal surgery have contributed to a higher incidence of these challenging cases worldwide.

Abdominal wall is a well-structured construction of skin, subcutaneous fat tissues, several muscle layers, preperitoneal fascia, and peritoneum, thus abdominal wall surgeons must deal with these different tissues mastering also reconstructive plastic surgery techniques [1].

1.2 Definition

There is no universally accepted definition of what constitutes a "CAW defect" [2, 3]. Some effort has been made to characterize factors of complexity associated with:

D. Cuccurullo (✉)
Unit of General, Laparoscopic and Robotic Surgery, A.O.R.N. dei Colli Monaldi Hospital, Naples, Italy
e-mail: diego.cuccurullo@ospedalideicolli.it

D. Cuccurullo, C. Rispoli (eds.), *Complex Abdominal Wall Surgery*, Updates in Surgery, https://doi.org/10.1007/978-3-032-24284-6_1

- Size and location
- Contamination and soft tissue condition
- Patient history
- Clinical scenario

These complexity factors are able to turn a simple hernia repair into a CAW reconstruction [4]. However, not all the features can be considered equal in characterizing complexity as some have a greater impact:

- Size of the defect: large defects, generally >10 cm in width, or those involving significant dimensions compared to abdominal morphology.
- Loss of domain: where the volume of herniated viscera exceeds 20–25% of the abdominal cavity or a ventral hernia large enough such that simple reduction in its contents and primary fascial closure cannot be achieved without additional reconstructive techniques or cannot be achieved without significant risk of complications due to the raised intra-abdominal pressure [5]. These patients need a really tailored approach with extensive use of prehabilitation strategies.
- Multiple recurrences: patients who have undergone several failed repairs, with distorted anatomy, scar tissue and meshes [6].
- Contamination or infection: presence of mesh infection, chronic wound infection, or enterocutaneous fistulas. Infections are a well-known factor affecting the morbidity, mortality and costs of surgery; consequently, the presence of a contaminated field creates a particularly challenging context for surgeries that are intended to be performed in clean conditions [7–9].
- Associated stomas or fistulas: parastomal hernias and fistula-associated defects. This condition represents one of the hardest to deal with, being a permanent stoma, a natural "hole" in the abdominal wall that should be addressed thoroughly.
- Severe comorbidities: including obesity, diabetes, immunosuppression, and pulmonary or cardiac disease.

These elements often overlap, reinforcing the need for individualized, multidisciplinary planning. The concept of complexity extends beyond the anatomical defect, encompassing systemic implications and the overall burden on the patient [10].

My personal definition of "a complex abdomen", always called "abdominal disaster" is driven mainly by this concept:

- Relevant damage of the abdominal wall, post-surgical, often with a "iatrogenic" contribution,
- With serious cardiovascular, respiratory, metabolic, skin impairments,
- Which involves local infections, aesthetic, psychological and social life impact,
- Not always solvable…
- And which, for its possible resolution, requires competence, experience, patience, availability of all "devices" and strategic planning,
- With, sometimes, planned, multiple interventions,

– And where proper preparation management may be the key to treatment.

In such complex cases, what many surgeons believe involves the closure of the fascia at the midline, often with reinforcement using mesh prosthetics is...simplistic.

Recurrence rates increase logarithmically, with 23.8% after the first reoperation, 35.3% after the second reoperation, and 38.7% after the third reoperation, so that any further surgery becomes more complex and hazardous [11].

1.3 Epidemiology

Even though new protocols for fascia closure have been developed and adopted worldwide [12, 13], abdominal wall closure often leads to failure.

Abdominal wall defects, particularly incisional hernias, represent one of the most frequent long-term complications of abdominal surgery. Their incidence ranges from 10% to 20% after midline laparotomy, with higher rates reported in high-risk groups (immunosuppressed, obese, malnourished, elderly patients or those with wound infection and any medical condition that is associated with an increase in intra-abdominal pressure in the postoperative period) [14].

The global rise in obesity and the increasing frequency of abdominal surgery for cancer and emergency conditions are major contributors to the growing burden of abdominal wall defects. Furthermore, improved survival of critically ill patients has led to more cases of open abdomen management, often resulting in large and complex hernias.

Patients who have undergone transplantation, vascular surgery and stoma creation represent a heterogeneous group that often will develop a CAW defect during their lifetime.

In the U.S.A., 4–5 million laparotomies are done annually, suggesting that at least 400,000–500,000 incisional hernias can be expected to occur every year. According to 2010 data, about 348,000 operations for incisional hernia are done every year in the U.S.A., with $3.2 billion in annual associated costs; estimates suggest that for every 1% reduction in ventral hernia rates in the U.S.A. there would be a $32 million cost-saving [15]. More recent data (2013) suggest an increase in these numbers: 611,000 operations per year with an estimated annual cost of $9.7 billion. The same 1% decrease in ventral hernia rates could save at least $139.9 million annually according to these more recent findings [16]. In some cases, incarceration and strangulation will lead to emergency surgery with increased costs and associated morbidity and mortality.

In this scenario, largely driven by the available means, lies the exorbitant cost of CAW reconstruction, whose cost can even increase tenfold when complications, ICU stay, and the multiple devices and procedures required are accounted for.

1.4 Clinical Relevance

The clinical impact of CAW defects extends far beyond the anatomical abnormality.

- Functional impairment: patients experience pain, impaired mobility, postural problems, and respiratory compromise in cases of large defects or loss of domain, often worsening pulmonary conditions.
- Systemic implications: malnutrition, altered pulmonary mechanics, and recurrent infections can significantly reduce physiological reserve.
- Psychological burden: disfigurement, loss of self-esteem, depression, and social isolation are frequently reported.
- Quality of life (QoL): numerous studies have demonstrated substantial impairment in health-related QoL, often comparable to chronic debilitating diseases.
- Economic impact: these conditions are associated with prolonged hospital stays, multiple reoperations, increased risk of complications, and a high cost to healthcare systems. Indirectly, they contribute to loss of productivity and long-term disability.

Functional impairment represents one of the most immediate and clinically relevant consequences, as patients commonly experience chronic pain, reduced mobility, postural alterations, and, in the presence of large defects or loss of domain, varying degrees of respiratory compromise, which may further exacerbate pre-existing pulmonary conditions. These local manifestations are frequently accompanied by systemic implications, including malnutrition, altered pulmonary mechanics, and recurrent cutaneous infectious episodes, all of which contribute to a significant reduction in physiological reserve and overall resilience to surgical stress. As a consequence of this global frailty, such patients are frequently deemed poor or unsuitable candidates for surgical treatment of concomitant diseases, leading to the under-treatment or delayed management of otherwise potentially operable conditions. Beyond the physical dimension, the psychological burden of these conditions is substantial: disfigurement and functional limitation often lead to loss of self-esteem, depressive symptoms, and progressive social isolation, further amplifying morbidity. Consistently, numerous clinical studies have demonstrated a marked deterioration in health-related QoL, with reported scores frequently comparable to those observed in chronic, severely debilitating diseases. Surgery is the only treatment for this severe impairment in QoL, with higher scores in operated patients compared to controls [17]. From a socioeconomic perspective, these conditions are associated with prolonged hospitalizations, repeated surgical interventions; indirectly, they also result in reduced work capacity, loss of productivity, and long-term disability.

Thus, CAW surgery should not be viewed solely as a technical procedure but rather as a comprehensive therapeutic pathway that addresses the patient's global health, functional recovery, and social reintegration.

1.5 Conclusion

CAW surgery has become a cornerstone of modern surgical practice, reflecting the intersection of technical innovation, multidisciplinary care, and patient-centered outcomes. The challenges associated with these conditions underscore the importance of specialized referral centers, evidence-based protocols, and continuous innovation in surgical techniques and biomaterials [18].

This book will explore the multiple dimensions of CAW surgery, from pathophysiology and clinical assessment to open, laparoscopic, and robotic repair strategies, as well as perioperative management and long-term outcomes.

An extensive description will be given of the major risk factors (immunosuppression, extreme obesity, malnutrition and any medical condition that is associated with increased intra-abdominal pressure) and their management.

Ultimately, the aim is to provide a comprehensive framework that supports surgeons worldwide in addressing one of the most demanding and impactful areas of contemporary surgery.

References

1. Lineaweaver WC. Abdominal wall reconstruction and patient comorbidities. Ann Plast Surg. 2018;81(1):1–2.
2. Latifi R, Gogna S. Surgery for complex abdominal wall defects: update of a nine-step treatment strategy. Surg Technol Int. 2022;40.sti40/1557.
3. Rosen MJ, editor. Atlas of abdominal wall reconstruction. 2nd ed. Philadelphia: Elsevier; 2017.
4. Slater NJ, Montgomery A, Berrevoet F, et al. Criteria for definition of a complex abdominal wall hernia. Hernia. 2014;18(1):7–17.
5. Parker SG, Halligan S, Liang MK, et al. Definitions for loss of domain: an international Delphi consensus of expert surgeons. World J Surg. 2020;44(4):1070–8.
6. Schoel LJ, Sinamo J, Williams J, et al. Heterogeneity in the surgical approach to recurrent abdominal wall hernias: an opportunity for quality improvement. Surg Endosc. 2024;38(11):6901–7.
7. Anderson DJ. Surgical site infections. Infect Dis Clin N Am. 2011;25(1):135–53.
8. Engemann JJ, Carmeli Y, Cosgrove SE, et al. Adverse clinical and economic outcomes attributable to methicillin resistance among patients with Staphylococcus aureus surgical site infection. Clin Infect Dis. 2003;36(5):592–8.
9. Atema JJ, de Vries FE, Boermeester MA. Systematic review and meta-analysis of the repair of potentially contaminated and contaminated abdominal wall defects. Am J Surg. 2016;212(5):982–95.e1.
10. Muysoms FE, Miserez M, Berrevoet F, et al. Classification of primary and incisional abdominal wall hernias. Hernia. 2009;13(4):407–14.
11. Flum DR, Horvath K, Koepsell T. Have outcomes of incisional hernia repair improved with time? A population-based analysis. Ann Surg. 2003;237(1):129–35.
12. Deerenberg EB, Harlaar JJ, Steyerberg EW, et al. Small bites versus large bites for closure of abdominal midline incisions (STITCH): a double-blind, multicentre, randomised controlled trial. Lancet. 2015;386(10000):1254–60.
13. Deerenberg EB, Henriksen NA, Antoniou GA, et al. Updated guideline for closure of abdominal wall incisions from the European and American Hernia Societies. Br J Surg. 2022;109(12):1239–50.

14. Helgstrand F, Rosenberg J, Kehlet H, et al. Nationwide prospective study of outcomes after elective incisional hernia repair. J Am Coll Surg. 2013;216(2):217–28.
15. Poulose BK, Shelton J, Phillips S, et al. Epidemiology and cost of ventral hernia repair: making the case for hernia research. Hernia. 2012;16(2):179–83.
16. Schlosser KA, Renshaw SM, Tamer RM, et al. Ventral hernia repair: an increasing burden affecting abdominal core health. Hernia. 2023;27(2):415–21.
17. Toma M, Oprea V, Scarlat F, et al. Quality of life and abdominal wall functionality after abdominal wall reconstruction: a prospective single center follow-up study. Hernia. 2024;28(6):2223–34.
18. Piccoli M, Agresta F, Attinà GM, et al. "Complex abdominal wall" management: evidence-based guidelines of the Italian consensus conference. Updat Surg. 2019;71(2):255–72.

Pathophysiology of Complex Abdominal Wall Defects and Systemic Implications

2

Biomechanical Alterations, Physiological Effects, and Impact on Patient Functions

Giuseppa Procida, Matteo Tolot, Alberto Grassetto, Paolo Lucernoni, Giulia Montori, and Ferdinando Agresta

2.1 Introduction

A complex abdominal wall defect is not simply a hernia but a multifaceted pathological state.

No clear and univocal definition emerges from the literature, but a recent Delphi consensus by the European Hernia Society has tried to give some answers [1].

A complex abdominal wall defect is characterized by many features such as massive size over 10 cm [1, 2], persistent or recurrent infections [2], exposed viscera, enterocutaneous fistulas, and significant lateral retraction of the abdominal wall musculature [3]. These defects are often the end-stage result of multiple prior surgical failures, abdominal catastrophes like necrotizing fasciitis, intra-abdominal sepsis or acute necrotizing pancreatitis, or the sequelae of damage control laparotomy [3].

Thus, a complex defect is defined less by its origin and more by its evolution into a condition that presents a profound therapeutic challenge to both the surgeon and the patient, often involving a history of complications and a high risk of future failure.

G. Procida (✉) · M. Tolot · G. Montori · F. Agresta
Department of General Surgery, Vittorio Veneto Hospital, AULSS2 Marca Trevigiana, Treviso, Italy
e-mail: giuseppa.procida@aulss2.veneto.it

A. Grassetto
Department of Anesthesiology, Vittorio Veneto Hospital, AULSS2 Marca Trevigiana, Treviso, Italy

P. Lucernoni
Department of Pneumology, Vittorio Veneto Hospital, AULSS2 Marca Trevigiana, Treviso, Italy

D. Cuccurullo, C. Rispoli (eds.), *Complex Abdominal Wall Surgery*, Updates in Surgery, https://doi.org/10.1007/978-3-032-24284-6_2

2.2 The Pathophysiology of Abdominal Wall Disruption

The clinical manifestation of a complex abdominal wall defect is the endpoint of a cascade of failure that begins at the molecular level and culminates in the gross biomechanical collapse of the abdominal container. Understanding this progression is essential for appreciating why simple repairs fail and why advanced reconstructive strategies are necessary.

Most abdominal wall defects ensue from a loss of the mechanical integrity of abdominal wall structural tissue, whose etiology is complex and multifactorial [4, 5].

2.2.1 Pathophysiology of Primary Hernia

To date, smoking and genetic predisposition are proposed as the main risk factors for the formation of primary abdominal wall hernias.

According to several studies, an abnormal structure and metabolism of extracellular matrix (ECM) in connective tissue leads to a predisposition to abdominal wall hernia formation and recurrence [6, 7]. Moreover, although not yet clearly demonstrated, an association between abdominal aortic aneurysm and abdominal wall hernia has also been observed, supporting the hypothesis of a shared pathophysiological mechanism, likely attributable to an impaired connective tissue metabolism [8, 9].

In patients with direct inguinal hernia, the anterior rectus sheath appears to be thinner, to have a lower collagen and elastic content, together with a lower hydroxyproline-to-proline ratio; moreover, the transversalis fascia of these patients tends to have a lower amount of collagen—mostly immature—and a higher quantity of elastic fibers, as well as lower lysine hydroxylation. The entirety of these changes results in reduced collagen stability, and in a subsequent decrease in fascial resistance [6].

In addition, evidence suggests a reduced type I:III collagen ratio in the anterior rectus sheath, in the transversalis fascia, and in the hernia sac and skin of patients with hernia. Type III collagen predominates in the early phase of wound healing and is considered to be thinner and less mature, providing less tensile strength compared to type I collagen [7]: therefore, a predominance of type III collagen leads to collagen fibres with reduced diameter and increased structural disorganization [10].

Matrix-metalloproteinases (MMPs) are a subgroup of zinc metalloproteinases involved in ECM degradation. An increase in MMP-1, MMP-2 and MMP-9 levels has been documented in the blood plasma and transversalis fascia of patients with inguinal hernia compared to controls: this impairment leads to an enhancement of their collagenolytic activity. In contrast, tissue inhibitors of metalloproteinases (TIMPs), whose role consists of inhibiting MMPs in order to prevent excessive degradation of ECM, appear to be reduced in the transversalis fascia of patients with inguinal hernia compared to controls [11].

2.2.2 Pathophysiology of Secondary Hernia

Although risk factors such as smoking, diet, comorbidities (diabetes, obesity, aortic aneurysm, perioperative hypotension) and deep wound infection may contribute to the development of secondary or incisional hernia [10], surgical incision is the predisposing condition for such a condition. According to Franz, the development of an incisional hernia primarily results from impaired acute wound healing, whereby alterations in any of the four phases of this process—hemostasis, inflammation, fibroproliferation and scar remodeling—triggered during laparotomy may ultimately lead to hernia formation [5].

After incision, the classical inflammatory pathway is activated, and an early migration of neutrophils to the wound site, followed by the recruitment of macrophages, occurs: together, these cellular types release several growth factors and inflammatory mediators that sustain inflammation and activate fibroblasts and MMPs [5, 10]. It has been shown that the loss of mechanical integrity of the abdominal wall drives the selection of an abnormal population of fibroblasts, associated with the secretion of altered collagen phenotype and a consistent decrease in the type I:III collagen ratio. This, in turn, results in early wound failure after laparotomy [10].

According to Thankam et al., the inflammation and ECM dysregulation induce the expression and activation of transforming growth factor-β1 (TGF-β1), which primarily activates TIMPs, thus inhibiting MMPs, and leads to an increase in type I:III collagen ratio. The ultimate result of this cascade is the differentiation of fibroblasts to myofibroblasts, a key event in the wound healing process. Furthermore, high-mobility group box 1 (HMGB1), a damage-associated molecular pattern molecule that activates the nuclear factor kappa-light-chain-enhancer of activated B cells (NFκB)-mediated release of TGF-β1, appears to contribute to this differentiation process. According to the authors, a reduced TGF-β1:HMGB1 ratio may therefore favor impaired wound healing, thereby promoting the development of incisional hernia [10].

2.3 Biomechanical Alterations

Abdominal wall hernia is the result of biochemical and biomechanical alterations. As previously discussed, alterations in the ECM result in weaker fascial tissue, which in turn predisposes to the development of wall defects [6].

Patients with incisional hernia have reduced abdominal wall dynamics due to altered function of abdominal wall core muscles [12, 13]. According to Sánchez Arteaga et al., their peak force generation capacity is approximately 20% lower than healthy controls, affecting both the rectus abdominis muscles and the lateral abdominal musculature; moreover, they show lower force generations rates. Male sex, larger hernia dimensions and elevated BMI appear to be the most influential factors contributing to the reduction of peak force [12].

2.4 The Concept of Loss of Domain

As the biomechanical failure of the abdominal wall progresses, it can reach a state known as "loss of domain" (LOD). This is the central pathophysiological concept in complex hernia surgery and the hallmark of the most challenging cases. However, the term has been plagued by the lack of a standardized definition, which has significantly hampered clinical research and the development of evidence-based treatment protocols [14].

Historically, LOD has been described with a variety of evocative but imprecise conceptual phrases. These include the notion of viscera having lost their "right of domain" or "right of domicile" within the abdomen, or the hernia sac enlarging to the point where it functions as a "second abdomen" [8]. While these descriptions capture the essence of the problem, their subjectivity limits their utility for scientific comparison [14]. In an effort to bring objectivity, quantitative definitions based on cross-sectional imaging have been proposed. These methods calculate the volume of the herniated viscera and compare it to the volume of the remaining intra-abdominal cavity. Yet, even here, inconsistency reigns [14, 15].

The two most cited methods, the Tanaka and Sabbagh methods, use different denominators for their calculations:

- The Tanaka method calculates the ratio of the hernia sac volume (HSV) to the abdominal cavity volume (ACV). The formula is LOD = HSV/ACV [16].
- The Sabbagh method calculates the ratio of the HSV to the total peritoneal volume (TPV), where TPV is the sum of the HSV and the ACV. The formula is LOD = HSV/(ACV + HSV) = HSV/TPV [17].

A "clinically significant" LOD is often cited at a threshold of >20% [17, 18], but this is largely based on anecdotal experience rather than rigorous data, and the specific method used is frequently not stated [14]. Without a universally accepted standard for what constitutes LOD, it is impossible to compare outcomes between studies, conduct meaningful meta-analyses, or develop high-level evidence-based guidelines for managing this patient population.

Regardless of the precise definition used, the core pathophysiology of LOD is the same: the chronic extrusion of abdominal viscera leads to a secondary, adaptive contraction of the "true" abdominal cavity. The abdominal wall musculature retracts laterally, the diaphragm assumes a more caudal position, and the peritoneal space shrinks [19]. The abdominal cavity effectively recalibrates to a smaller volume.

2.5 Systemic Implications and Multi-organ Dysfunction

The chronic disruption of the abdominal wall and the acute stress of surgical repair trigger physiological changes like inflammation and sudden hemodynamic shifts that affect organs including the lungs, heart, visceral and genitourinary system.

These effects underlie the widespread, multi-organ consequences of both the disease process and its treatment. Consequently, the pathophysiology of complex abdominal wall defect reflects that of a systemic disease.

2.5.1 Respiratory Compromise: Chronic to Acute

A large complex abdominal wall defect impacts the respiratory system in both its chronic unrepaired condition and during the acute period following surgical correction. In the chronic state of LOD, the abdominal wall loses its tone and ability to provide counter-pressure to the diaphragm. This allows the diaphragm to descend to a lower, flatter, and less efficient position. The normal synergistic, piston-like action of the thoracoabdominal cylinder is lost, replaced by a state of chronic incoordination between the chest wall, diaphragm, and atrophied abdominal muscles. The primary physiological consequence is a marked decrease in chest wall compliance. To achieve adequate ventilation against this stiffened chest wall, the patient must expend significantly more energy, leading to an increase in the mechanical work of breathing and greater oxygen consumption by the respiratory muscles. This can result in a state of latent chronic respiratory failure, where the patient may experience dyspnea on exertion but have deceptively normal spirometry and blood gas analysis at rest [20].

Surgical repair of the wall defect transforms this chronic dysfunction into an acute crisis. The reduction of herniated viscera into a smaller abdominal cavity results in a rapid and sometimes significant increase in intra-abdominal pressure (IAP). The increased pressure pushes forcefully against the diaphragm, limiting its movement. The lungs, now compressed from below, have reduced functional residual capacity and compliance. This acute physiological insult can precipitate postoperative respiratory failure, making it difficult or impossible to wean the patient from mechanical ventilation. The risk of atelectasis and subsequent pneumonia or pleural effusion or exacerbation of a known COPD/bronchial asthma is markedly increased. In its most extreme form, the uncontrolled rise in IAP can lead to abdominal compartment syndrome, a life-threatening condition of multi-organ failure driven by critically impaired perfusion [21].

An important role in these pathological events is also played by the difficulty in coughing and the damage to mucociliary clearance which can occur in the immediate postoperative period for the reasons already indicated and primarily for postoperative pain [22].

This highlights a crucial paradox: the definitive surgical treatment for the chronic disease is itself the trigger for the most acute and life-threatening respiratory complications.

2.5.2 Strategies to Reduce Postoperative Respiratory Complications

A. **General Measures**

1. Smoking cessation: Preferably at least 8 weeks prior to surgery. Shorter cessation periods may still be beneficial and should be encouraged, as they can provide non-respiratory advantages [23].
2. Optimization of pre-existing respiratory conditions, such as COPD or bronchial asthma. All efforts should be made to discontinue oral corticosteroids.
3. Proper treatment of infectious symptoms and ensuring adequate recovery time after resolution. Following influenza, COVID-19, or lower respiratory tract bacterial infections, a minimum waiting period of two weeks is recommended, which may extend up to seven weeks in the case of severe infections.
4. Preoperative dental evaluation or sanitation, or at least preventive dental assessment.
5. Preoperative cycle of pulmonary rehabilitation, especially in high-risk patients with chronic bronchopulmonary diseases (e.g., COPD) [24]. The rehabilitation program should include aerobic training and exercises to strengthen respiratory muscles, and should last no less than two weeks. Its efficacy should be evaluated through repeat spirometry and functional tests. All patients should be trained and educated in postoperative pulmonary rehabilitation techniques, including incentive spirometry [25].
6. Restrict the use of antibiotics to only prophylaxis protocols against surgical wound infection.

B. **Intraoperative Measures**

1. Prefer shorter surgical procedures, ideally under three hours [26].
2. Pulmonary recruitment [27].
3. Consider alternatives to general anesthesia, including neuraxial anesthesia or regional analgesia.
4. Use β-adrenergic bronchodilators prior to intubation in patients with obstructive pulmonary diseases.
5. During general anesthesia, apply low tidal volumes (e.g., 6–8 mL/kg) and a positive end-expiratory pressure (PEEP) of 6–8 cm H_2O [27].
6. Avoid long-acting neuromuscular blocking agents during induction and maintenance, and ensure proper reversal of muscle relaxation at the end of the procedure.

C. **Postoperative Measures**

1. Use non-invasive ventilation support techniques when needed.
2. Apply respiratory physiotherapy techniques that promote lung expansion and routinely use incentive spirometry [25].

3. Encourage early mobilization of the patient [23].
4. Ensure adequate pain control, preferably using epidural analgesia. Be cautious with opioids and avoid NSAIDs in asthmatic patients.
5. Avoid routine use of nasogastric tubes owing to the risk of aspiration.
6. Prevent venous thromboembolism.
7. Implement appropriate pharmacological mucolysis, particularly in patients with excessive bronchial secretions (e.g., bronchiectasis) [23].

2.5.3 Cardiovascular Effects: Direct and Indirect

The cardiovascular system is also placed under severe strain by large hernias and their repair. While direct cardiac compression is a well-documented phenomenon in giant hiatal hernias, where the herniated stomach can physically impinge on the left atrium and ventricle, causing tamponade physiology and arrhythmias like atrial fibrillation [28], similar hemodynamic instability can occur indirectly by the repair of a large ventral hernia with LOD.

The mechanism is the acute rise in IAP and a consequent intra-abdominal hypertension (IAH), which is defined by a sustained or repeated pathological elevation in IAP $\geq$12 mmHg [29].

The elevated pressure within the abdomen can compress the inferior vena cava, drastically impeding venous return to the heart. This reduction in preload can lead to a sharp drop in cardiac output and profound hemodynamic instability. Furthermore, the massive fluid shifts that can occur during the dissection and reduction of a giant hernia sac contribute to this instability [30].

A striking case report documented a 73-year-old man undergoing repair of a giant inguinoscrotal hernia who experienced severe intraoperative cardiovascular collapse. Following reduction of the hernia contents and abdominal closure, he developed new-onset atrial fibrillation with a rapid ventricular response and went into cardiorespiratory arrest. This case demonstrates that the acute physiological insult of reversing LOD can mimic the hemodynamic effects of direct cardiac compression, posing a significant risk of life-threatening cardiovascular events [31].

2.5.4 Visceral and Genitourinary System Alterations

The organs contained within the hernia sac, as well as those in the adjacent genitourinary system, are subject to both chronic and acute pathological changes.

The viscera that reside chronically outside the abdominal cavity undergo significant adaptation. Due to the constant dependent position and potential kinking of vessels at the hernia neck, venous and lymphatic return from the mesentery is impaired. This leads to chronic mesenteric edema, thickening, and elongation. The bowel loops themselves, having lost the normal counter-pressure of the abdominal wall (a phenomenon known as loss of visceral-parietal tonus), can become chronically dilated and hypomotile. The skin overlying a massive hernia is often stretched thin, atrophic, and poorly vascularized, making it susceptible to pressure sores, ulceration, and the formation of enterocutaneous fistulas.

The urinary system also can be affected; it could be directly involved in the hernia itself. Herniation of the urinary bladder occurs in 1–3% of all inguinal hernias [32]. While many are asymptomatic, patients may present with lower urinary tract symptoms (LUTS) such as dysuria, frequency, urgency, or nocturia. The pathognomonic sign is "two-stage micturition", where the patient first voids the intra-abdominal portion of the bladder, and then must manually compress the hernia to empty the herniated portion. A groin mass with LUTS should raise suspicion for bladder involvement.

More rarely, the ureter can herniate, typically into the inguinal canal. This can lead to kinking and obstructive uropathy with resultant hydronephrosis, a critical consideration in any patient with an inguinal hernia and unexplained renal dysfunction, particularly those with a history of renal transplantation [33]. Inadvertent injury to a herniated and unrecognized bladder or ureter is a major surgical risk, which underscores the importance of preoperative imaging in any patient with a suspicious presentation. Finally, even when the urinary tract is not directly involved in the hernia, hernia repair surgery itself is a significant risk factor for postoperative urinary retention (POUR). Affecting 5–25% of patients, POUR is caused by a combination of anesthetic effects, opioid analgesia, and local surgical inflammation interfering with normal bladder sensation and function [34].

Acute kidney dysfunction can instead be observed following surgical repair of a voluminous abdominal hernia with LOD, with the same pathogenetic mechanism that underlies cardiovascular disorders—i.e., a rapid and sustained increase in IAP with consequent reduction of venous return, renal hypoperfusion and therefore acute kidney injury (AKI) [29].

2.5.5 Musculoskeletal Changes and Functional Loss

The abdominal wall is the central component of the body's core, providing the stable base for posture and movement. The biomechanical failure inherent in a complex abdominal wall defect leads to progressive core muscle weakness. This loss of anterior support has downstream consequences for the entire musculoskeletal frame. The spine, now lacking its anterior tension band, is subjected to abnormal forces, which can lead to deleterious changes in lumbar lordosis and the development of chronic, debilitating back pain. Patients with incisional hernias demonstrate significantly reduced abdominal muscle strength and overall physical performance, which contributes to a marked decline in their health-related quality of life (HRQoL) scores, particularly in domains related to physical functioning [35].

2.6 Quality of Life and Psychological Impact

Beyond the measurable organ dysfunction, the most profound systemic implication of a complex abdominal wall defect is its devastating impact on the patient's life and sense of self. Patients suffer from a range of physical symptoms, including chronic pain, which can be a dull ache or sharp and activity-related, discomfort from the sheer weight and bulk of the hernia, swelling, and associated gastrointestinal and urinary issues.

However, these symptoms have major psychological and social consequences. Qualitative research has revealed the deep psychological toll of living with a large hernia. Patients report significantly higher rates of low mood, depression, and anxiety.

This loss of identity can lead to social withdrawal, fear of judgment, and the development of complex psychological coping mechanisms. This psychological burden is not merely an outcome of the disease; it is an integral part of its pathophysiology. There is a plausible feedback loop wherein the psychological distress, through neuroendocrine pathways (e.g., chronic stress and cortisol elevation), may further impair wound healing and immune function, thus exacerbating the underlying biological drivers of the disease. This makes the assessment and support of a patient's mental health an integral part of managing their complex systemic disease state [36].

Table 2.1 summarizes the clinical consequences, and the underlying pathophysiological mechanism, of a complex abdominal wall defect and its surgical correction.

Table 2.1 Systemic consequences of complex abdominal wall defects

Organ system	Chronic pathophysiological State (unrepaired)	Chronic clinical manifestations (unrepaired)	Acute pathophysiology of repair	Acute clinical manifestations of repair
Respiratory	Low/inefficient diaphragm; Decreased chest wall compliance; Muscle incoordination	Dyspnea on exertion; Latent respiratory insufficiency; Paradoxical respiratory motion	Sudden increase in IAP; Diaphragmatic splinting; Decreased lung compliance	Acute respiratory failure; Ventilator dependence; Pneumonia; Abdominal compartment syndrome
Cardiovascular	Potential for hemodynamic adaptation to altered pressures	Generally stable in chronic state, unless direct compression occurs (rare in ventral hernias)	Sudden increase in IAP; Impeded venous return (IVC compression); Massive fluid shifts	Hemodynamic instability/collapse; Arrhythmias (e.g., atrial fibrillation); Cardiorespiratory arrest
Gastrointestinal/Visceral	Mesenteric edema/thickening; Chronic bowel dilatation; Impaired motility	Chronic discomfort; Poor bowel function; Risk of ulceration, fistula, incarceration/strangulation	Reduction of chronically adapted viscera; Potential for ischemic injury during dissection	Ileus; Bowel injury; Risk of ACS-related bowel ischemia
Genitourinary	Direct herniation of bladder/ureter; Chronic bladder outlet obstruction	LUTS (frequency, urgency); Two-stage micturition; Obstructive uropathy/hydronephrosis	Risk of iatrogenic injury to herniated structures during repair; Anesthetic/analgesic effects on bladder function	Bladder/ureter injury; Postoperative urinary retention; Acute kidney injury (due to IAH)
Musculoskeletal	Loss of core muscle integrity; Chronic muscle unloading, atrophy, and fibrosis	Chronic back pain; Altered spinal curvature; Decreased strength and physical function	Re-tensioning of atrophied muscles; Closure under tension	Postoperative pain; Potential for fascial dehiscence or recurrence if tension is excessive
Psychological/QoL	Chronic pain/discomfort; Negative body image; Social withdrawal	Depression; Anxiety; Loss of identity; Severely impaired quality of life	Stress of major surgery; Fear of complications and recurrence	Postoperative delirium; Anxiety about recovery and long-term outcome

ACS abdominal compartment syndrome, *IAH* intra-abdominal hypertension, *IAP* intra-abdominal pressure, *IVC* inferior vena cava, *LUTS* lower urinary tract symptoms, *QoL* quality of life

References

1. Capoccia Giovannini S, Podda M, Ribas S, et al. What defines an incisional hernia as 'complex': results from a Delphi consensus endorsed by the European Hernia Society (EHS). Br J Surg. 2024;111(1):znad346.
2. Slater NJ, Montgomery A, Berrevoet F, et al. Criteria for definition of a complex abdominal wall hernia. Hernia. 2014;18(1):7–17.
3. Turégano F, García-Marín A. The biology of complex abdominal wall defects: definitions and causes. In: Latifi R, editor. Surgery of complex abdominal wall defects. 1st ed. New York: Springer; 2013. p. 15–23.
4. Jansen PL, Mertens Pr PR, Klinge U, Schumpelick V. The biology of hernia formation. Surgery. 2004;136(1):1–4.
5. Franz MG. The biology of hernias and the abdominal wall. Hernia. 2006;10(6):462–71.
6. Henriksen NA, Yadete DH, Sorensen LT, et al. Connective tissue alteration in abdominal wall hernia. Br J Surg. 2011;98(2):210–9.
7. Harrison B, Sanniec K, Janis JE. Collagenopathies – implications for abdominal wall reconstruction: a systematic review. Plast Reconstr Surg Glob Open. 2016;4(10):e1036.
8. Hall KA, Peters B, Smyth SH, et al. Abdominal wall hernias in patients with abdominal aortic aneurysmal versus aortoiliac occlusive disease. Am J Surg. 1995;170(6):572–5.
9. Antoniou GA, Georgiadis GS, Antoniou SA, et al. Abdominal aortic aneurysm and abdominal wall hernia as manifestations of a connective tissue disorder. J Vasc Surg. 2011;54(4):1175–81.
10. Thankam FG, Palanikumar G, Fitzgibbons RJ, Agrawal DK. Molecular mechanisms and potential therapeutic targets in incisional hernia. J Surg Res. 2019;236:134–43.
11. Bracale U, Peltrini R, Iacone B, et al. A systematic review on the role of matrix metalloproteinases in the pathogenesis of inguinal hernias. Biomolecules. 2023;13(7):1123.
12. Sánchez Arteaga A, Gil Delgado JL, Feria Madueño A, et al. Impact of incisional hernia on abdominal wall strength. BJS Open. 2024;8(3):zrae045.
13. Roy NB, Khan WF, Krishna A, et al. A comparative study to evaluate abdominal wall dynamics in patients with incisional hernia compared to healthy controls. Surg Endosc. 2023;37(12):9414–9.
14. Parker SG, Halligan S, Blackburn S, et al. what exactly is meant by "loss of domain" for ventral hernia? Systematic review of definitions. World J Surg. 2019;43(2):396–404.
15. Parker SG, Halligan S, Liang MK, et al. Definitions for loss of domain: an international Delphi consensus of expert surgeons. World J Surg. 2020;44(4):1070–8.
16. Tanaka EY, Yoo JH, Rodrigues AJ Jr, et al. A computerized tomography scan method for calculating the hernia sac and abdominal cavity volume in complex large incisional hernia with loss of domain. Hernia. 2010;14(1):63–9.
17. Sabbagh C, Dumont F, Robert B, et al. Peritoneal volume is predictive of tension-free fascia closure of large incisional hernias with loss of domain: a prospective study. Hernia. 2011;15(5):559–65.
18. Bueno-Lledó J, Torregrosa A, Jiménez R, et al. Preoperative combination of progressive pneumoperitoneum and botulinum toxin type A in patients with loss of domain hernia. Surg Endosc. 2018;32(8):3599–608.
19. Parikh KR, Al-Hawary M, Millet JD, et al. Incisional hernia repair: what the radiologist needs to know. AJR Am J Roentgenol. 2017;209(6):1239–46.
20. De Santis L, Frigo F, Bruttocao A, Terranova O. Pathophysiology of giant incisional hernias with loss of abdominal wall substance. Acta Biomed. 2003;74(Suppl 2):34–7.
21. Van Hoef S, Dries P, Allaeys M, et al. Intra-abdominal hypertension and compartment syndrome after complex hernia repair. Hernia. 2024;28(3):701–9.
22. Piccioni F, Spagnesi L, Pelosi P, et al. Postoperative pulmonary complications and mortality after major abdominal surgery. An observational multicenter prospective study. Minerva Anestesiol. 2023;89(11):964–76.

23. Chandler D, Mosieri C, Kallurkar A, et al. Perioperative strategies for the reduction of postoperative pulmonary complications. Best Pract Res Clin Anaesthesiol. 2020;34(2):153–66.
24. Fernandes A, Rodrigues J, Lages P, et al. Root causes and outcomes of postoperative pulmonary complications after abdominal surgery: a retrospective observational cohort study. Patient Saf Surg. 2019;13:40.
25. do Nascimento Junior P, Módolo NSP, Andrade S, et al. Incentive spirometry for prevention of postoperative pulmonary complications in upper abdominal surgery. Cochrane Database Syst Rev. 2014;2014(2):CD006058.
26. Ashraf N, Zargar OU, Albina A, Ahmed S. Study of incidence and factors associated with postoperative pulmonary complications in patients undergoing abdominal surgery. Int J Res Med Sci. 2024;12(11):4129–35.
27. Pei S, Wei W, Yang K, et al. Recruitment maneuver to reduce postoperative pulmonary complications after laparoscopic abdominal surgery: a systematic review and meta-analysis. J Clin Med. 2022;11(19):5841.
28. Gnanenthiran SR, Naoum C, Kilborn MJ, Yiannikas J. Posterior cardiac compression from a large hiatal hernia – a novel cause of ventricular tachycardia. HeartRhythm Case Rep. 2018;4(8):362–6.
29. Kirkpatrick AW, Roberts DJ, De Waele J, et al. Intra-abdominal hypertension and the abdominal compartment syndrome: updated consensus definitions and clinical practice guidelines from the World Society of the Abdominal Compartment Syndrome. Intensive Care Med. 2013;39(7):1190–206.
30. Carmona-Puerta R, Pérez-Sanchez D, Pichardo-Ureña JM, et al. The cardiovascular effects of large hiatal hernias: a narrative review of cases and studies. Postgrad Med. 2024;136(4):358–65.
31. Hever P, Dhar M, Cavale N. Loss of domain leading to intra-operative cardiorespiratory arrest during open repair of a giant inguinoscrotal hernia and hydrocele. JPRAS Open. 2018;16:1–5.
32. Elkbuli A, Narvel RI, McKenney M, Boneva D. Inguinal bladder hernia: a case report and literature review. Int J Surg Case Rep. 2019;58:208–11.
33. Eilber KS, Freedland SJ, Rajfer J. Obstructive uropathy secondary to ureteroinguinal herniation. Rev Urol. 2001;3(Fall 4):207–8.
34. Blair AB, Dwarakanath A, Mehta A, et al. Postoperative urinary retention after inguinal hernia repair: a single institution experience. Hernia. 2017;21(6):895–900.
35. van Ramshorst GH, Eker HH, Hop WCJ, et al. Impact of incisional hernia on health-related quality of life and body image: a prospective cohort study. Am J Surg. 2012;204(2):144–50.
36. Smith OA, Mierzwinski MF, Chitsabesan P, Chintapatla S. Health-related quality of life in abdominal wall hernia: let's ask patients what matters to them? Hernia. 2022;26(3):795–808.

Preoperative Planning and Risk Stratification

3

Ernesto Tartaglia

3.1 Introduction

Complex abdominal wall reconstruction (AWR) presents a formidable challenge in general surgery, characterized by a high incidence of postoperative complications. The paradigm for managing these patients has evolved from a primarily technical focus to one emphasizing comprehensive preoperative planning and physiological optimization. Evidence conclusively demonstrates that outcomes are significantly influenced by patient-specific factors identifiable and modifiable before intervention [1]. This chapter provides a structured framework for the preoperative assessment and risk stratification of patients undergoing complex AWR. The objective is to equip the surgeon with a systematic methodology to reduce modifiable risks, accurately predict surgical challenges, and formulate a data-driven operative plan, thereby converting a high-risk procedure into a controlled, strategic intervention.

3.2 Comprehensive Patient Assessment

The journey toward a successful reconstruction begins with a first clinical encounter that is less a simple consultation and more a comprehensive investigative session. This initial assessment is designed to gather the raw data—both subjective and objective—that will inform every subsequent decision, from the timing of surgery to the specific technical approach taken in the operating room.

E. Tartaglia (✉)
Unit of General, Laparoscopic and Robotic Surgery, A.O.R.N. dei Colli Monaldi Hospital, Naples, Italy
e-mail: ernesto.tartaglia@gmail.com

D. Cuccurullo, C. Rispoli (eds.), *Complex Abdominal Wall Surgery*, Updates in Surgery, https://doi.org/10.1007/978-3-032-24284-6_3

3.2.1 Clinical History and Physical Examination

Taking a history for complex AWR requires a methodical and almost narrative approach, seeking to understand the full story of the patient's abdominal wall. It is imperative to document the origin event—be it a prior surgical incision, trauma, or infection—and to trace the hernia's evolution over time, noting its progression, any previous attempts at repair—surgical techniques, mesh types employed, and any history of wound complications or prosthetic infection—and the specific circumstances of any failures, which often hold the key to avoiding future complications [2]. The patient's symptom profile must be thoroughly elucidated, distinguishing between simple cosmetic concerns, visceral pressure, previous or actual site infection, episodes of incarceration, and debilitating pain that may suggest nerve entrapment or mesh-related issues. Concurrently, a detailed review of systems is crucial to paint a complete picture of the patient's physiological landscape; uncontrolled COPD or chronic heart failure can dramatically increase intra-abdominal pressure and compromise healing, while diabetes mellitus and immunocompromised states directly impair cellular repair mechanisms and immune defense. The physical examination then serves to ground this historical information in tangible reality. It involves a careful topographic mapping of the abdominal wall, palpating the borders of the defect, assessing the integrity and tone of the lateral musculature, and evaluating the quality and pliability of the overlying soft tissue. The presence of multiple scars, thin skin, or a large, dependent pannus that creates a chronic intertriginous environment is not merely an observation but a critical data point that may dictate the need for concurrent panniculectomy or collaboration with a plastic surgeon to ensure a robust soft tissue closure [3].

3.2.2 Preoperative Imaging

Cross-sectional imaging with computed tomography (CT) constitutes an indispensable component of the preoperative assessment for complex AWR, providing critical quantitative data that fundamentally informs surgical decision-making and operative strategy [4]. Modern imaging protocols mandate multiphase acquisition including thin-slice axial, coronal, and sagittal reconstructions. The inclusion of provocative maneuvers, particularly the acquisition of images during a patient-executed Valsalva maneuver, is essential as it enables dynamic assessment of fascial integrity, reveals occult or intermittent herniations, and permits accurate quantification of true hernia dimensions under physiological conditions of elevated intra-abdominal pressure.

The diagnostic utility of preoperative CT extends beyond mere anatomical documentation to enable precise morphometric and volumetric analysis that directly correlates with surgical complexity and postoperative risk. Key analytical applications include (Table 3.1):

Table 3.1 Key metrics obtainable from preoperative CT imaging

Metric	Description	Clinical significance
Defect width	Largest transverse diameter on axial imaging	Defects >10 cm typically necessitate component separation techniques [6]
Loss of domain ratio	(Herniated content volume/total peritoneal volume) × 100	Ratio >20–25% indicates need for preoperative expansion strategies [5]
Rectus muscle width	Midline to linea semilunaris distance	Predicts medial advancement capacity post-component separation [7]
Subcutaneous fat thickness	Skin-to-fascia distance at midline	Depth >2–3 cm constitutes independent risk factor for wound morbidity [8]

- Hernia defect morphometry: Precise measurement of the maximum transverse fascial defect diameter is a critical determinant for establishing the necessity and type of component separation techniques required to achieve tension-free medialization of the myofascial layers [5].
- Quantification of loss of domain (LOD): Calculated volumetrically as (hernia sac volume/total peritoneal volume) × 100. An LOD ratio exceeding 20–25% indicates a significant reduction in functional abdominal domain and visceral accommodation, often necessitating consideration of advanced preoperative strategies such as botulinum toxin A injections into the lateral abdominal wall muscles or progressive preoperative pneumoperitoneum to facilitate fascial coaptation and mitigate respiratory compromise [6].
- Myofascial architecture analysis: Measurement of rectus muscle width and lateral abdominal wall thickness provides predictive information regarding the potential for medial advancement following anterior or posterior component separation techniques, which is vital for procedural planning [7]. For example, the Rives-Stoppa technique alone is enough when the sum of the bilateral rectus muscle width is at least twice the maximal defect width—confirming Carbonell's algorithm, presented at the 9th Annual Abdominal Wall Reconstruction Summit, Montana US, 2018: additional myofascial release (transversus abdominis release, TAR) may be necessary if the maximal defect width closely approximates or exceeds twice the rectus width.
- Soft tissue composition assessment: Quantification of subcutaneous adipose tissue depth, particularly when exceeding 2–3 cm, has been consistently demonstrated as an independent risk factor for wound morbidity and surgical site occurrences, thereby influencing decisions regarding surgical approach, incision placement, and closure methodology [8].

3.3 Risk Stratification and Optimization

The process of risk stratification is the analytical engine of preoperative planning, where collected data is synthesized into a coherent risk profile. This is not a passive exercise in labeling patients as "high-risk", but an active and dynamic process of identifying vulnerabilities and implementing targeted interventions to fortify the patient against potential complications. By objectively categorizing patient risk, surgeons can make informed decisions about whether to proceed with surgery, which surgical strategy to adopt, and how best to prepare the patient.

3.3.1 Optimizing Modifiable Risk Factors

This critical phase focuses on the malleable aspects of a patient's physiology, representing the surgeon's most powerful opportunity to alter the postoperative trajectory.

Smoking cessation stands as a non-negotiable prerequisite; the toxic effects of nicotine-induced vasoconstriction and tissue hypoxia, combined with the impaired neutrophil function caused by other cigarette components, create a wound environment hostile to healing and profoundly increase the risk of mesh infection and fascial dehiscence. A minimum abstinence period of four weeks, verified objectively through serum cotinine testing, is considered essential to begin reversing this pathophysiology [9].

Obesity presents, as well, a multifactorial challenge that often must be addressed before considering elective repair. A BMI exceeding 40 kg/m^2 is associated with exponentially increased rates of surgical site occurrences, as the thick, poorly vascularized subcutaneous panniculus impedes oxygen delivery and serves as a potential space for fluid collection, while the associated chronic state of inflammation and mechanically elevated intra-abdominal pressure places immense strain on any repair. Therefore, a referral for supervised medical or surgical weight loss is not a dismissal of the patient but a necessary first step in a responsible surgical journey, with a target BMI of 35 or below representing a benchmark that has consistently been shown to dramatically improve outcomes [10, 11].

Glycemic control is another pillar of optimization; an elevated glycosylated hemoglobin (HbA_{1c}) is a marker of a dysmetabolic state that impairs immune cell function and collagen synthesis. Collaborating with an endocrinologist to achieve an HbA_{1c} below 7.0% for a sustained period prior to surgery is a standard evidence-based practice to reduce infectious complications [12].

Finally, the *assessment of nutritional status* moves beyond a simple albumin check; it is an evaluation of the body's metabolic capacity to heal. Hypoalbuminemia signifies a catabolic state incapable of mounting the anabolic response required for successful wound healing and integration of a prosthetic material. Preoperative supplementation with high-protein, high-calorie nutritional shakes or, in severe cases, delaying surgery for formal enteral or parenteral nutrition, is a therapeutic intervention as important as any antibiotic prophylaxis [13].

3.3.2 Risk Prediction Tools

Several tools are available. The European Hernia Society (EHS) classification, introduced to standardize reporting of primary and incisional abdominal wall hernias, is highly practical when applied to preoperative planning [14]. It codifies

Table 3.2 European Hernia Society incisional hernia classification

Midline	Subxiphoidal		M1
	Epigastric		M2
	Umbilical		M3
	Infraumbilical		M4
	Suprapubic		M5
Lateral	Subcostal		L1
	Flank		L2
	Iliac		L3
	Lumbar		L4
Recurrent incisional hernia?		Yes ☐ No ☐	
Length: cm		**Width**: cm	
Width cm	W1 <4 cm ☐	W2 ≥4–10 cm ☐	W3 ≥10 cm ☐

anatomical localization and transverse width using simple, reproducible categories—information that directly affects technical choices in the operating room. The EHS incisional hernia classification is summarized in Table 3.2.

The American Society of Anesthesiologists (ASA) score remains a universal standard for assessing anesthetic risk and overall fitness for surgery. While not specific to hernia repair, it provides a baseline stratification that correlates with morbidity and mortality [15].

The Ventral Hernia Working Group (VHWG) classification has particular relevance, as it accounts for both the degree of wound contamination and the presence of comorbidities. The VHWG introduced the term "surgical site occurrence" (SSO) as a comprehensive umbrella term to encompass all perioperative wound events, thereby providing a more complete picture of postoperative morbidity than surgical site infection (SSI) alone [1]. This classification includes:

- Infection, which can be subclassified according to the Centers for Disease Control criteria as superficial, deep, or organ space SSI [16]. It is critical to note that wound cellulitis not requiring incision manipulation is classified as an SSO, not an SSI.
- Sterile fluid collections, such as seromas or hematomas.
- Wound dehiscence.
- Enterocutaneous fistulae, including enteroprosthetic fistulae.

In its 2010 guidelines, the VHWG also developed a grading system designed to predict the risk of SSO and SSI, which is summarized in Table 3.3 [1].

Subsequent validation efforts by Kanters et al. in 2012 led to a critical refinement of this system [17]. Their analysis revealed that immunosuppression was not a statistically significant predictor of SSO and should not be included as a Grade 2 comorbidity. Furthermore, they found no significant difference in SSO rates between Grade 2 and Grade 3 patients, or between Grade 3 and Grade 4 patients. Specifically, comorbid Grade 2 patients had SSO rates similar to Grade 3 patients with a history

Table 3.3 Ventral Hernia Working Group grading system

Grade 1	Grade 2	Grade 3	Grade 4
Low risk	*Comorbid*	*Potentially contaminated*	*Infected*
Low risk of complications No history of wound infection	Smoking Obesity Diabetes Immunosuppression	Prior wound infection Presence of ostomy Violation of the gastrointestinal tract	Grossly infected mesh Septic dehiscence

Table 3.4 Modified Ventral Hernia Working Group grading system

Grade 1	Grade 2	Grade 3
Low risk	*Comorbid*	*Contaminated*
Low risk of complications No history of wound infection	Smoking Obesity Diabetes Immunosuppression Prior wound infection	Clean-contaminated Contaminated Active infection
SSO = 14%	SSO = 27%	SSO = 46%

SSO surgical site occurrence

of prior wound infection, while other Grade 3 patients had rates akin to infected Grade 4 cases. These findings prompted a modified classification that reclassifies prior wound infection as a Grade 2 risk factor and combines the former Grade 3 and 4 categories into a single "contaminated" tier (Table 3.4) [17].

While instrumental, both the original and modified VHWG systems have been critiqued for excluding several important patient, hernia, and operative variables. Factors such as acute incarceration, concomitant procedures, operative time, and the extent of dissection are not accounted for in these models.

To address this, Berger and colleagues proposed the Ventral Hernia Risk Score (VHRS), a points-based system derived from the odds ratios of variables most strongly associated with SSO/SSI, specifically for open ventral hernia repair (Table 3.5) [18]. This model represents a more nuanced, albeit complex, approach to risk stratification.

In a parallel effort to standardize the definition of a "complex" abdominal wall hernia, Slater et al. (2013) convened a consensus group to establish criteria based on both opinion and evidence [19]. They identified and categorized key variables into four domains (Patient, Hernia, Contamination, and Surgical history) and further proposed three patient severity classes—Minor, Moderate, and Major—to reflect the anticipated need for escalating perioperative resources, postoperative complexity, and financial cost (Tables 3.6 and 3.7) [19]. This framework aims to improve comparative outcomes research across studies and techniques. The critical next step is the development and validation of treatment algorithms that can guide the selection of surgical technique and prosthetic material based on these stratified risk profiles.

The Carolinas Equation for Determining Associated Risks (CeDAR) score represents a more sophisticated tool, incorporating variables such as smoking, diabetes, and obesity to predict the likelihood of wound-related complications [20].

By amalgamating variables like BMI, defect size, history of surgical site infection, and comorbid conditions, these tools generate a quantitative, personalized risk estimate for complications and recurrence. It can be particularly useful in preoperative discussions with patients, helping them understand the importance of risk modification, and can also rationally guide technical choices.

Table 3.5 Ventral Hernia Risk Score for surgical site occurrence and surgical site infection

	VHRS for SSO			VHRS for SSI		
Variable	OR	95% CI	Points	OR	95% CI	Points
Mesh implant	1.9	1.4–2.7	2	–	–	–
Concomitant hernia repair	2.2	1.5–3.4	2	2.1	1.4–3.3	2
Skin flaps created	2.2	1.6–3.1	2	2.3	1.6–3.4	2
ASA score ≥3	–	–	–	2.1	1.4–3.2	2
BMI ≥40	–	–	–	3.2	1.7–5.9	3
Wound class 4	8.7	3.7–24.1	9	6.8	3.2–15.4	7

ASA American Society of Anesthesiologists, *BMI* body mass index, *OR* odds ratio, *SSO* surgical site occurrence, *SSI* surgical site infection, *VHRS* Ventral Hernia Risk Score

Table 3.6 Criteria for definition of a complex abdominal wall hernia (patient)

1. Size and location
Large-sized abdominal wall hernia, ≥10 cm in width
Parastomal, lumbar, lateral and subcostal locations of hernias
Loss of domain ≥20%
2. Contamination and soft tissue condition
Wound environment with surgical wound class III ('Contaminated') or IV ('Dirty')
Full-thickness abdominal wall defects
Loss of substance (e.g., after tumor resection, trauma, infection)
Distorted anatomy (e.g., after multiple previous procedures)
Denervated muscles
Skin grafts
Wound ulcers/non-healing wound
Open abdomen
Disease related (omphalocele, necrotizing fasciitis)
Presence of enterocutaneous fistula
3. Patient history and risk factors
Recurrent hernia after an earlier mesh repair or component separation
Comorbidities/risk factors that impair wound healing: obesity, diabetes, old age, steroid use, or poor nutritional state (albumin <30 g/dL)
Increased intra-abdominal pressure: obesity, COPD
Previous wound dehiscence
Previous mesh infection
4. Clinical scenario
Emergency operation with bowel resection
Intraperitoneal mesh removal
Multiple hernia defects (e.g., 'battle-scarred abdomen')
No primary closure possible without component separation

COPD chronic obstructive pulmonary disease

Table 3.7 Complex hernia criteria grouped in the patient severity classes 'Minor', 'Moderate' and 'Major' dependent upon expected increase in peri-operative measures and planning, risk of complications, and costs

Minor	Moderate	Major
Only one wound healing impairing risk factor[a]	Two or more wound healing impairing risk factors[a] Hernia >10 cm in width, or no primary closure possible without component separation Loss of domain >20% Parastomal, lumbar, lateral and subcostal hernias Full-thickness defects, loss of substance, distorted anatomy or multiple hernia defects Skin grafts, wound ulcers, non-healing wound Disease related: omphalocele Increased intra-abdominal pressure: COPD, obesity History of wound dehiscence or wound/mesh infection Intraperitoneal mesh removal Emergency operation with bowel resection	Two or more wound healing impairing risk factors[a] and one or more 'Moderate' class criteria Surgical wound class III ("Contaminated") or IV ("Dirty") Open (burst) abdomen Disease related: necrotizing fasciitis Current mesh infection Enterocutaneous fistula present

[a]Obesity, diabetes, steroid use, smoking, old age, poor nutritional state (albumin <30 g/dl)
COPD chronic obstructive pulmonary disease

3.4 The Multidisciplinary Team Approach

The inherent complexity of these patients definitively shatters the model of the surgeon as a solitary operator. Achieving excellence in complex AWR is now recognized as the product of a coordinated, multidisciplinary enterprise, a "pit crew" approach where each specialist contributes their expertise to prepare the patient for the operative event. The anesthesiologist's role begins preoperatively, conducting a thorough assessment of cardiopulmonary function and orchestrating a multimodal analgesic plan that emphasizes regional blocks (e.g., transversus abdominis plane blocks) to minimize opioid consumption and its attendant risks of ileus and respiratory depression. The nutritionist or dietician provides the rigorous, evidence-based dietary intervention needed to correct protein-calorie deficits and build metabolic reserve. For the morbidly obese patient, the bariatrician becomes an essential partner, guiding and monitoring significant weight loss, which is often the single most effective risk-reduction strategy available [10, 11]. Furthermore, the physical therapist plays a crucial role in preoperative education, teaching patients breathing techniques to strengthen their respiratory drive and instructing them on the mechanics of log-rolling and protected movement to safeguard the repair post-operatively. This collaborative ecosystem ensures that the patient presented for surgery is not merely "cleared" but is actively optimized, with every member of the care team aligned toward a common goal of achieving a durable and uncomplicated recovery.

3.5 Surgical Strategy Planning

The data gathered preoperatively directly informs the operative plan:

- Technique selection: Decision between open, laparoscopic, robotic or hybrid approach; planning for various component separation techniques (e.g., posterior versus anterior, endoscopic versus open) [6, 21–24].
- Mesh considerations: Choice of mesh type (synthetic, biosynthetic, biologic), weight, and position (onlay, retromuscular, preperitoneal, intraperitoneal) based on patient risk factors and contamination level (e.g., Ventral Hernia Working Group grade) [1, 25].
- Adjunct procedures: Planning for potential panniculectomy, ostomy reversal, or collaboration with plastic surgery for soft tissue reconstruction [3].

3.6 Conclusion

In conclusion, the management of complex abdominal wall hernias has been fundamentally redefined. The surgeon's expertise is now demonstrated not first with a scalpel but through the intellectual rigor of preoperative planning and the disciplined management of patient optimization. This chapter has outlined a comprehensive framework for this process, underscoring that a successful outcome is the product of a meticulous, multi-stage preparation that integrates detailed anatomical mapping with profound physiological insight. By embracing a philosophy that prioritizes risk stratification and modification, and by leveraging the collective strength of a multidisciplinary team, surgeons can effectively de-escalate the inherent risks of these formidable procedures. This deliberate and holistic approach allows for the creation of a truly personalized surgical plan, turning the operating room into a venue for the execution of a strategy forged through weeks or months of careful preparation. Ultimately, the greatest testament to surgical skill in the twenty-first century may be the recognition that the path to a durable, functional, and safe AWR is paved long before the patient is ever positioned on the operating table.

References

1. Ventral Hernia Working Group, Breuing K, Butler CE, et al. Incisional ventral hernias: review of the literature and recommendations regarding the grading and technique of repair. Surgery. 2010;148(3):544–58.
2. Petro CC, Rosen MJ. A current review of long-acting resorbable meshes in abdominal wall reconstruction. Plast Reconstr Surg. 2018;142(3 Suppl):84S–91S.

3. Fischer JP, Basta MN, Wink JD, et al. Optimizing patient selection in ventral hernia repair with concurrent panniculectomy: an analysis of 1974 patients from the ACS-NSQIP datasets. J Plast Reconstr Aesthet Surg. 2014;67(11):1532–40.
4. Aguirre DA, Santosa AC, Casola G, Sirlin CB. Abdominal wall hernias: imaging features, complications, and diagnostic pitfalls at multi-detector row CT. Radiographics. 2005;25(6):1501–20.
5. Novitsky YW, Elliott HL, Orenstein SB, Rosen MJ. Transversus abdominis muscle release: a novel approach to posterior component separation during complex abdominal wall reconstruction. Am J Surg. 2012;204(5):709–16.
6. Tanaka EY, Yoo JH, Rodrigues AJ Jr, et al. A computerized tomography scan method for calculating the hernia sac and abdominal cavity volume in complex large incisional hernia with loss of domain. Hernia. 2010;14(1):63–9.
7. Miller BT, Ellis RC, Petro C, et al. Quantitative tension on the abdominal wall in posterior components separation with transversus abdominis release. JAMA Surg. 2023;158(12):1321–6.
8. Love MW, Warren JA, Davis S, et al. Computed tomography imaging in ventral hernia repair: can we predict the need for myofascial release? Hernia. 2021;25(2):471–7.
9. Sørensen LT. Wound healing and infection in surgery: the pathophysiological impact of smoking, smoking cessation, and nicotine replacement therapy: a systematic review. Ann Surg. 2012;255(6):1069–79.
10. Prabhu AS, Dickens EO, Copper CM, et al. Laparoscopic vs robotic intraperitoneal mesh repair for incisional hernia: an Americas Hernia Society quality collaborative analysis. J Am Coll Surg. 2017;225(2):285–93.
11. Liang MK, Holihan JL, Itani K, et al. Ventral hernia management: expert consensus guided by systematic review. Ann Surg. 2017;265(1):80–9.
12. Martindale RG, Deveney CW. Preoperative risk reduction: strategies to optimize outcomes. Surg Clin North Am. 2013;93(5):1041–55.
13. Weimann A, Braga M, Carli F, et al. ESPEN guideline: clinical nutrition in surgery. Clin Nutr. 2017;36(3):623–50.
14. Muysoms FE, Miserez M, Berrevoet F, et al. Classification of primary and incisional abdominal wall hernias. Hernia. 2009;13(4):407–14.
15. Wolters U, Wolf T, Stützer H, Schröder T. ASA classification and perioperative variables as predictors of postoperative outcome. Br J Anaesth. 1996;77(2):217–22.
16. Horan TC, Gaynes RP, Martone WJ, et al. CDC definitions of nosocomial surgical site infections, 1992: a modification of CDC definitions of surgical wound infections. Infect Control Hosp Epidemiol. 1992;13(10):606–8.
17. Kanters AE, Krpata DM, Blatnik JA, et al. Modified hernia grading scale to stratify surgical site occurrence after open ventral hernia repairs. J Am Coll Surg. 2012;215(6):787–93.
18. Berger RL, Li LT, Hicks SC, et al. Development and validation of a risk-stratification score for surgical site occurrence and surgical site infection after open ventral hernia repair. J Am Coll Surg. 2013;217(6):974–82.
19. Slater NJ, Montgomery A, Berrevoet F, et al. Criteria for definition of a complex abdominal wall hernia. Hernia. 2014;18(1):7–17.
20. Plymale MA, Davenport DL, Walsh-Blackmore S, et al. Costs and complications associated with infected mesh for ventral hernia repair. Surg Infect (Larchmt). 2020;21(4):344–9.
21. Bittner R, Bain K, Bansal VK, et al. Update of Guidelines for laparoscopic treatment of ventral and incisional abdominal wall hernias (International Endohernia Society (IEHS)) – Part A. Surg Endosc. 2019;33(10):3069–139.
22. Sagnelli C, Tartaglia E, Guerriero L, et al. Long-term outcomes of Madrid approach after TAR for complex abdominal wall hernias: a single-center cohort study. Hernia. 2024;28(3):769–77.

23. Cuccurullo D, Guerriero L, Mazzoni G, et al. Robotic transabdominal retromuscular rectus diastasis (r-TARRD) repair: a new approach. Hernia. 2022;26(6):1501–9.
24. Rognoni C, Cuccurullo D, Borsoi L, et al. Clinical outcomes and quality of life associated with the use of a biosynthetic mesh for complex ventral hernia repair: analysis of the "Italian Hernia Club" registry. Sci Rep. 2020;10(1):10706.
25. Carbonell AM, Criss CN, Cobb WS, et al. Outcomes of synthetic mesh in contaminated ventral hernia repairs. J Am Coll Surg. 2013;217(6):991–8.

4 Prehabilitation in Complex Abdominal Wall Surgery: Nutritional, Respiratory, and Physical Conditioning Strategies

Frederik Berrevoet, Anton Jult, and Pieter Dries

4.1 Introduction

Primary ventral and incisional hernia repair is among the most common abdominal wall procedures performed by general surgeons worldwide [1]. Postoperative consequences differ depending on the cause and surgical method, ranging from low-risk primary hernia repair to sophisticated abdominal wall reconstruction [2, 3]. Because most repairs require the implantation of a synthetic or (long-term) resorbable mesh, reducing wound complications is critical to avoid long-term recurrence [4, 5]. Aside from the clinical implications, complications following hernia surgery significantly raise healthcare expenditures and reduce patient-reported quality of life [6, 7].

Prehabilitation, or the adjustment of physical, nutritional, and psychological state before surgery, has been shown to reduce postoperative morbidity in vascular, colorectal, bariatric, hepatic, and urologic surgeries [8]. Most hernias are benign, allowing for attentive waiting, which provides an important chance to improve controllable risk variables before elective treatment [9]. Exercise-based therapies have demonstrated safety and efficacy in improving muscle function and cardiopulmonary fitness prior to bariatric, cardiovascular, and orthopedic surgeries [10]. However, evidence for prehabilitation prior to abdominal wall reconstruction is still limited, but appears to be growing.

Patients with extensive ventral hernias form a separate patient subgroup, frequently presenting with decreased movement, respiratory constraint, and pain due to the abdominal wall defect. These conditions not only diminish quality of life, but also limit physical activity and raise the likelihood of incarceration. Despite technological breakthroughs in open, laparoscopic, and robotic techniques, with or

F. Berrevoet (✉) · A. Jult · P. Dries
Department for General and HPB Surgery and Liver Transplantation,
Ghent University Hospital, Ghent, Belgium
e-mail: frederik.berrevoet@ugent.be; anton.jult@uzgent.be; dries.pieter@gmail.com

D. Cuccurullo, C. Rispoli (eds.), *Complex Abdominal Wall Surgery*, Updates in Surgery, https://doi.org/10.1007/978-3-032-24284-6_4

without mesh implantation, recurrence rates can still reach 30% [1–5]. Surgical site complications (e.g., infection, seroma, hematoma) occur in 10–60% of cases, depending on patient and hernia heterogeneity [6]. Such issues lengthen hospital stays, increase readmission rates, and raise resource consumption [7].

Recent research has shown prehabilitation as a viable technique for addressing these issues, increasing functional reserve, and reducing surgical stress [8]. Multimodal programs that combine fitness training, dietary counseling and psychological support have been shown to increase postoperative recovery in thoracic, esophagogastric, and colorectal cancer populations [9–13]. Nonetheless, the research clearly indicates risk factors for poor outcomes in complex hernia repair, although evidence for the usefulness of prehabilitation in ventral or incisional hernia surgery is limited [14–19].

4.2 Nutrition

Nutritional status is a critical factor in wound healing and surgical recovery. Malnutrition and sarcopenic obesity are linked to poor results during abdominal wall repair. A thorough search revealed no studies that directly assessed preoperative dietary optimization in ventral hernia repair [20]. Indirect data from colorectal and oncologic surgery suggests that preoperative dietary guidance and protein supplementation can minimize morbidity. Nutritional prehabilitation could thus be included into hernia optimization paths through proven evaluation techniques and customized supplements.

4.3 Weight Loss Interventions

4.3.1 Non-surgical Weight Loss

The research on preoperative dietary weight loss prior to ventral hernia repair contains only a few trials. One study found that implementing a low-calorie diet (~458 kcal/day) in morbidly obese patients (mean BMI 44 kg/m^2) resulted in a weight loss of approximately 15% of the starting body weight, lowering BMI to around 37 kg/m^2 [20]. In a study of 20 patients, Goldberg et al. found that either an 800 kcal meal replacement or a 1200 kcal restricted diet resulted in a mean weight loss of around 9.8% [21]. Plymale et al. analyzed registry data and found that patients who achieved a preoperative weight-loss goal had better outcomes [22], while a cohort of patients with BMI > 35 kg/m^2 achieved an 18% BMI reduction via a protein-sparing fast (~800 kcal/day) and maintained weight loss in 88% of patients at 18 months [23]. Although first approved for the treatment of type 2 diabetes, glucagon-like peptide 1 (GLP-1) receptor agonists have moved into the mainstream as pharmacologic adjuncts for weight loss, with established safety and efficacy in both diabetic and non-diabetic individuals [24]. There is a growing body of literature investigating the utility of GLP-1 agonists as a tool for perioperative weight management in surgical patients, and Spurzem et al. demonstrated in a recent study that GLP-1 agonists accelerate preoperative weight loss in obese hernia patients without negatively impacting postoperative outcomes [25]. These studies show practicality and safety in chosen patients, but randomized data are insufficient, and the results are strongly dependent on motivation and multidisciplinary support.

4.3.2 Operative Weight Loss Interventions

Several studies have reported outcomes when bariatric surgery is performed before hernia repair. The staged approach appears to reduce wound complications and recurrence, particularly in patients with large or complex hernias. Laparoscopic sleeve gastrectomy is preferred due to a lesser risk of abdominal wall problems and faster weight loss. Recently, Rodriguez-Gonçalves and colleagues showed in their retrospective analysis that bariatric surgery patients had both the highest initial weight (116.9 kg) and BMI (42.8 kg/m^2), followed by the pharmacotherapy group (99.1 kg, 37.9 kg/m^2) and the dietary counseling group (95.0 kg, 35.5 kg/m^2), but they also accomplished the greatest weight reduction, with a mean loss of 20.7% (SD: 15.5), compared with 4.6% (SD: 6.0) in the dietary counseling group and 4.4% (SD: 3.5) in the pharmacotherapy group ($p < 0.001$). BMI reductions followed a similar pattern [26]. However, difficulties remained widespread, highlighting the need for personalized, interdisciplinary prehabilitation techniques. As a result, it appears worthwhile to pursue bariatric surgery in higher BMI groups before pursuing elective and more difficult abdominal wall reconstructions.

4.4 Physical Therapy

Physical training is an important component of multimodal prehabilitation, although data for abdominal wall rebuilding remain sparse. To date, only two randomized controlled trials have evaluated preoperative physical therapy in patients having ventral hernia surgery, both of which reported on the same research cohort at separate time periods [8, 27].

Bernardi et al. conducted the initial short-term examination of a prehabilitation program for obese patients scheduled for elective ventral hernia surgery, comparing an educational and home-based exercise intervention to conventional care. Although the intervention group showed a minor reduction in 30-day wound complications—specifically a lower seroma incidence—there were no statistically significant differences in overall morbidity, functional recovery, or quality of life. The same group's subsequent long-term research revealed no sustained improvement in recurrence rates after 2 years (27.1% in the exercise group vs. 33.9% in controls). Interestingly, the prehabilitation cohort had a greater rate of early conversion to emergency repair, but this could have been due to random variation given the small sample size. The physical activity component was mostly made up of unsupervised home-based exercises such as aerobic, stretching, and resistance-band training, supplemented by instructional materials rather than in-person physiotherapy. The lack of a structured, supervised exercise component most likely reduced the intervention's efficacy.

A systematic analysis published in 2021 found that procedures for ventral hernia repair are not routinely performed, and it highlighted the rationale and practicality of physical therapy as a routine practice in ventral hernia repair [28]. Early functional rehabilitation is a pillar of therapy in tendon reconstruction, as well as fascial reconstruction during hernia surgery, and it is crucial for favorable outcomes with early mobilization. Similarly, rehabilitation in the first few months after hernia repair is most likely critical for preventing hernia recurrence, improving function, reducing pain through non-pharmacological therapy, improving patient well-being, and decreasing fatigue. In a study of 275 patients, Pezeshk et al. [29] found that a systematic rehabilitation program reduced ventral hernia recurrence rates from 22% to 9% ($p < 0.01$) over 5 years.

Although the total evidence is ambiguous, the findings indicate that unsupervised physical activity guidance is insufficient to improve surgical outcomes in this population. Future studies should look into professionally supervised, customized exercise regimens that focus on core stability, cardiovascular fitness, and mobility, ideally integrated into larger multimodal prehabilitation protocols.

4.5 Smoking Cessation

Smoking is a well-known independent risk factor for postoperative wound problems, poor mesh integration, and hernia recurrence following open incisional hernia repair. Furthermore, active smokers had a higher risk of pulmonary morbidity, delayed healing, and chronic pain after abdominal surgery [30, 31].

Gronkjoer et al. conducted a comprehensive review and meta-analysis of 107 papers examining the impact of smoking on postoperative complications in all types of surgical intervention. Tobacco usage enhanced the likelihood of overall morbidity, wound, infectious, pulmonary, and neurologic problems [32].

Sørensen et al. studied 344 patients undergoing open inguinal or incisional hernia surgery and exposed them to various smoking cessation treatments [33]. Patients who received formal cessation counseling had considerably greater abstinence rates than controls (19% vs. 2%), especially when reinforced by outpatient classes and telephone follow-up. Although there was no statistically significant difference in wound complications (7% vs. 5%), the trend supported the intervention. They also conducted a meta-analysis of over 480,000 patients across several subspecialties and discovered that smoking was associated with higher risks of wound dehiscence, surgical site infection, and subsequent hernia formation [34]. A randomized controlled experiment conducted by the same group found that smokers were more likely to develop a wound complication. Interestingly, this study also found that quitting smoking for 4 weeks produced results comparable to people who had never smoked [35]. In a separate study, they found that smokers were four times more likely to develop an incisional hernia following abdominal surgery [36]. In ventral hernia repair, major investigations from the Veterans Health Administration facilities and the National Surgical Quality Improvement Program database revealed that smokers had greater incidence of wound infections, including superficial, deep, and organ space infections. This elevated risk, however, can be mitigated and eventually reversed with at least 4 weeks of preoperative abstinence [37, 38].

Møller et al. conducted a randomized controlled experiment on 117 patients undergoing primary hernia repair, laparoscopic cholecystectomy, or orthopedic surgery. They provided extensive smoking cessation counseling and nicotine replacement for 4 weeks before and after surgery [39]. The intervention group had a much lower postoperative complication rate than the controls (21% vs. 41%), resulting in a 49% relative risk reduction.

Holland et al. have established a route to execute preoperative smoking cessation and diabetes control for at least 4 weeks [40]. All diabetic and smoking patients were given the same preoperative advice on the importance of blood glucose management, exercise, weight loss, and smoking cessation. A positive cotinine test would cancel the procedure. Following preoperative smoking cessation, the majority of smoking patients (58.6%) continued to abstain from tobacco use at their most recent follow-up. Alternatively, just 14.9% of non-optimized patients stopped smoking after surgery on their own. They demonstrated that improved diabetic control and smoking cessation minimize morbidity associated with these comorbidities to the same level as non-diabetic and non-smoking patients.

In clean patients, data from the Abdominal Core Health Quality Collaborative revealed equal 30-day morbidity and surgical site infection rates in smokers and non-smokers [41]. They have subsequently discontinued requiring smoking cessation, although the same data indicated a significant drop in surgical site occurrence (12.0% vs. 7.4%; $p = 0.03$) and pneumonia (5.7% vs. 0.7%; $p = 0.01$) after quitting. While most research only looked at open abdominal wall reconstruction, this makes the conclusions less applicable to minimally invasive procedures. According to reports, open abdominal wall reconstruction patients who are preoptimized have similar outcomes as preoptimized robotic abdominal wall reconstruction patients [42].

Although specific data for ventral hernia repair remain sparse, these findings highlight the potential benefit of an organized, multidisciplinary smoking cessation program as part of prehabilitation. Preoperative smoking cessation programs, ideally starting at least 4 weeks before surgery, should be considered standard practice in abdominal wall reconstruction pathways.

4.6 Conclusions

In conclusion, prehabilitation and patient optimization prior to ventral and incisional hernia surgery are reasonable and increasingly evidence-based treatments [43]. Preoperative planning should include weight loss, exercise, dietary enhancement, and smoking cessation. This has also been demonstrated in recent studies on the effectiveness of using a prehabilitation pathway for ventral and incisional hernia repair [43]. Although high-quality hernia-specific trials are scarce, the implementation of structured optimization paths suited to the abdominal wall patient may improve surgical preparedness, reduce complications, and improve long-term results.

References

1. Burger JWA, Luijendijk RW, Hop WCJ, et al. Long-term follow-up of a randomized controlled trial of suture versus mesh repair of incisional hernia. Ann Surg. 2004;240(4):578–83.
2. Ehlers AP, Sinamo JK, Howard R, et al. Long-term risk of mesh infection requiring removal after elective ventral hernia repair. JAMA Surg. 2025;160(2):1318–25.
3. Deerenberg EB, Timmermans L, Hogerzeil DP, et al. A systematic review of the surgical treatment of large incisional hernia. Hernia. 2015;19(1):89–101.
4. Holihan JL, Nguyen DH, Nguyen MT, et al. Mesh location in open ventral hernia repair: a systematic review and network meta-analysis. World J Surg. 2016;40(1):89–99.
5. Jairam AP, Timmermans L, Eker HH, et al. Prevention of incisional hernia with prophylactic onlay and sublay mesh reinforcement versus primary suture only in midline laparotomies (PRIMA): 2-year follow-up of a multicentre, double-blind, randomised controlled trial. Lancet. 2017;390(10094):567–76.
6. de Jong DLC, Wegdam JA, Berkvens EHM, et al. Does quality of life improve after complex incisional hernia repair? A systematic review. Hernia. 2025;29(1):110.
7. Plymale MA, Davenport DL, Walsh-Blackmore S, et al. Costs and complications associated with infected mesh for ventral hernia repair. Surg Infect. 2020;21(4):344–9.
8. Liang MK, Bernardi K, Holihan JL, et al. Modifying risks in ventral hernia patients with prehabilitation: a randomized controlled trial. Ann Surg. 2018;268(4):674–80.
9. Minnella EM, Carli F. Prehabilitation and functional recovery for colorectal cancer patients. Eur J Surg Oncol. 2018;44(7):919–26.
10. Barberan-Garcia A, Ubré M, Roca J, et al. Personalised prehabilitation in high-risk patients undergoing elective major abdominal surgery: a randomized blinded controlled trial. Ann Surg. 2018;267(1):50–6.
11. Santa Mina D, Clarke H, Ritvo P, et al. Effect of total-body prehabilitation on postoperative outcomes: a systematic review and meta-analysis. Physiotherapy. 2014;100(3):196–207.
12. Bolger JC, Loughney L, Tully R, et al. Perioperative prehabilitation and rehabilitation in esophagogastric malignancies: a systematic review. Dis Esophagus. 2019;32(9):doz058.
13. Moran J, Guinan E, McCormick P, et al. The ability of prehabilitation to influence postoperative outcome after intra-abdominal operation: a systematic review and meta-analysis. Surgery. 2016;160(5):1189–201.
14. Cattaneo M, Jastaniah A, Ghezeljeh TN, et al. Effectiveness of prehabilitation for patients undergoing complex abdominal wall surgery. Surg Endosc. 2025;39(5):3364–72.
15. Martin D, Besson C, Pache B, et al. Feasibility of a prehabilitation program before major abdominal surgery: a pilot prospective study. J Int Med Res. 2021;49(11):3000605211060196.
16. de Jong DLC, Wegdam JA, Driessen ICM, et al. Exploring psychological prehabilitation in complex abdominal wall reconstruction: a prospective pilot study. J Abdom Wall Surg. 2025;4:15195.
17. McLurcan N, Sanders DL, Hollyman M, et al. Randomized controlled trials of weight loss before hernia surgery: a systematic review and meta-analysis. J Abdom Wall Surg. 2025;4:15234.
18. Findlay JM, Sanders DL. Tailoring weight loss before hernia surgery: distinguishing between two types of obesity. J Abdom Wall Surg. 2025;4:14322.
19. Kollias V, Reid J, Udayasiri D, et al. Towards a complete cycle of care: a multidisciplinary pathway to improve outcomes in complex abdominal wall hernia repair. ANZ J Surg. 2022;92(9):2025–36.

20. Jensen KK, East B, Jisova B, et al. The European Hernia Society prehabilitation project: a systematic review of patient prehabilitation prior to ventral hernia surgery. Hernia. 2022;26(3):715–26.
21. Goldberg RF, Parker M, Stauffer JA, et al. Surgeon's requirement for obesity reduction: its influence on weight loss. Am Surg. 2012;78(3):325–8.
22. Plymale MA, Davenport DL, Roth JS. Outcomes experienced by patients presenting with ventral hernia and morbid obesity in a surgical clinic. Am Surg. 2017;83(8):e344–6.
23. Rosen MJ, Aydogdu K, Grafmiller K, et al. A multidisciplinary approach to medical weight loss prior to complex abdominal wall reconstruction: is it feasible? J Gastrointest Surg. 2015;19(8):1399–406.
24. Ilanga M, Heard JC, McClintic J, et al. Use of GLP-1 agonists in high risk patients prior to bariatric surgery: a cohort study. Surg Endosc. 2023;37(12):9509–13.
25. Spurzem GJ, Broderick RC, Ruiz-Cota P, et al. The new bridge to hernia surgery: achieving preoperative weight optimization with GLP-1 receptor agonists for abdominal wall hernia repair. Surg Endosc. 2025;39(8):5296–302.
26. Rodrigues-Gonçalves V, Verdaguer-Tremolosa M, Martínez-López P, et al. Obesity-focused prehabilitation strategies in ventral hernia: cohort study. Hernia. 2025;29(1):202.
27. Bernardi K, Olavarria OA, Dhanani NH, et al. Two-year outcomes of prehabilitation among obese patients with ventral hernias: a randomized controlled trial (NCT02365194). Ann Surg. 2022;275(2):288–94.
28. Perez JE, Schmidt MA, Narvaez A, et al. Evolving concepts in ventral hernia repair and physical therapy: prehabilitation, rehabilitation, and analogies to tendon reconstruction. Hernia. 2021;25(4):1–13.
29. Pezeshk RA, Pulikkottil BJ, Mapula S, et al. Complex abdominal wall reconstruction: a novel approach to postoperative care using physical medicine and rehabilitation. Plast Reconstr Surg. 2015;136(3):362e–9e.
30. Gupta H, Gupta PK, Schuller D, et al. Development and validation of a risk calculator for predicting postoperative pneumonia. Mayo Clin Proc. 2013;88(11):1241–9.
31. Lode L, Oma E, Henriksen NA, Jensen KK. Enhanced recovery after abdominal wall reconstruction: a systematic review and meta-analysis. Surg Endosc. 2021;35(2):514–23.
32. Grønkjær M, Eliasen M, Skov-Ettrup LS, et al. Preoperative smoking status and postoperative complications: a systematic review and meta-analysis. Ann Surg. 2014;259(1):52–71.
33. Sorensen LT, Karlsmark T, Gottrup F. Abstinence from smoking reduces incisional wound infection: a randomized controlled trial. Ann Surg. 2003;238(1):1–5.
34. Sørensen LT. Wound healing and infection in surgery. The clinical impact of smoking and smoking cessation: a systematic review and meta-analysis. Arch Surg. 2012;147(4):373–83.
35. Sørensen LT, Jørgensen T. Short-term pre-operative smoking cessation intervention does not affect postoperative complications in colorectal surgery: a randomized clinical trial. Color Dis. 2003;5(4):347–52.
36. Sørensen LT, Hemmingsen U, Jørgensen T. Strategies of smoking cessation intervention before hernia surgery—effect on perioperative smoking behavior. Hernia. 2007;11(4):327–33.
37. Thomsen T, Villebro N, Møller AM. Interventions for preoperative smoking cessation. Cochrane Database Syst Rev. 2014;2014(3):CD002294.
38. Park H, de Virgilio C, Kim DY, et al. Effects of smoking and different BMI cutoff points on surgical site infection after elective open ventral hernia repair. Hernia. 2021;25(2):337–43.
39. Møller AM, Villebro N, Pedersen T, Tønnesen H. Effect of preoperative smoking cessation on postoperative complications: a randomised clinical trial. Lancet. 2002;359(9301):114–7.
40. Holland AM, Wiley AJ, Kerr SW, et al. The impact of preoperative optimization for abdominal wall reconstruction on long-term glucose control and smoking cessation. Surg Endosc. 2025;39(10):6742–51.
41. Fafaj A, de Figueiredo SMP, Rosen MJ, Petro CC. Preoperative optimization in hernia surgery: are we really helping or are we just stalling? Hernia. 2024;28(3):925–30.

42. Kerr SW, Lorenz WR, Holland AM, et al. Outcomes of open versus robotic preperitoneal ventral hernia repair: a propensity-matched analysis. Hernia. 2025;29(1):197.
43. Marcolin P, Poli M, de Figueiredo S, Walmir de Araújo S, et al. Preoperative optimization before ventral hernia repair: a systematic review and meta-analysis. Surg Laparosc Endosc Percutan Tech. 2023;33(2):211–8.

Surgical Anatomy of the Abdominal Wall

5

Pierre Gueroult, Paulo Barros, and Yohann Renard

5.1 Introduction

The term abdominal wall conveys a static idea of this structure and is probably inappropriate to describe a complex cylindrical structure involved in trunk mobility, respiration, expulsive movements such as defecation, coughing, and urination, and in the containment of intra-abdominal organs [1]. This complexity is also reflected at the anatomical level by the interweaving of several layers with distinct functions. From superficial to deep, these include the skin, the superficialis fascia, the subcutaneous tissue, the musculo-aponeurotic layers, the preperitoneal space, the transversalis fascia, and the parietal peritoneum.

The abdominal wall extends from the inferior part of the thorax to the superior part of the pelvis [2]. Laterally and posteriorly, it continues to the erector spinae muscles and the quadratus lumborum. It can therefore be divided into an anterior part, roughly hexagonal in shape, and a posterior part, which will be described separately.

Knowledge of the anatomy of the abdominal wall allows understanding of parietal pathologies but also of repair techniques and their specific difficulties.

In this chapter, we will successively describe the different layers of the anterior and posterior abdominal wall, their vascularization, and their innervation. Special attention will be given to the anterior abdominal wall, which represents the vast majority of repairs encountered by the surgeon.

P. Gueroult (✉) · Y. Renard
Department of General, Digestive and Endocrine Surgery, Robert-Debré University Hospital, University of Reims Champagne-Ardenne, Reims, France
e-mail: pgueroult@chu-reims.fr; yrenard@chu-reims.fr

P. Barros
Department of General Surgery, Hospital Israelita Albert Einstein, São Paulo, Brazil

D. Cuccurullo, C. Rispoli (eds.), *Complex Abdominal Wall Surgery*, Updates in Surgery, https://doi.org/10.1007/978-3-032-24284-6_5

5.2 Antero-Lateral Abdominal Wall

5.2.1 Superficial Layers

Three superficial structures can be distinguished: the skin, the subcutaneous tissue, and the superficialis fascia.

5.2.1.1 Skin

The skin of the anterior abdominal wall is relatively mobile compared with the musculo-aponeurotic plane (Fig. 5.1). It is anchored to the abdominal wall by the umbilicus, acting as a medial fixation point. Horizontal surface tension lines were described by Langer and correspond to the orientation of collagen fibers in the dermis [3]. Several folds are visible: a suprapubic fold in women, a subumbilical fold halfway between the umbilicus and the pubis, a supraumbilical fold, and a

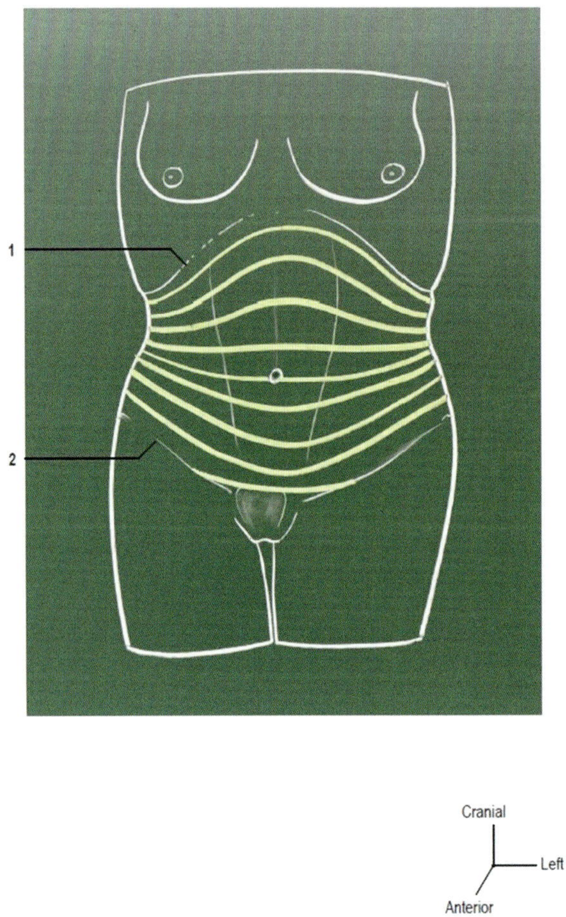

Fig. 5.1 Superficial anterior abdominal wall—Langer's lines. (1) Right costal margin; (2) Right Malgaigne line (right inguinal ligament)

cutaneous fold along the groin (Malgaigne line). Following these lines during abdominal incisions ensures an optimal cosmetic result [4].

5.2.1.2 Subcutaneous Tissue

This consists of adipose tissue with variable thickness depending on its location (Fig. 5.2). It is often thicker in its inferior part and may be responsible for a pendulous abdomen in obese patients. It is divided into two layers, superficial and deep, by the superficialis fascia. This tissue is poorly vascularized, which, during wide subcutaneous dissections, may cause wound dehiscence and skin necrosis.

5.2.2 Muscles

The muscles of the abdominal wall are arranged in different orientations.

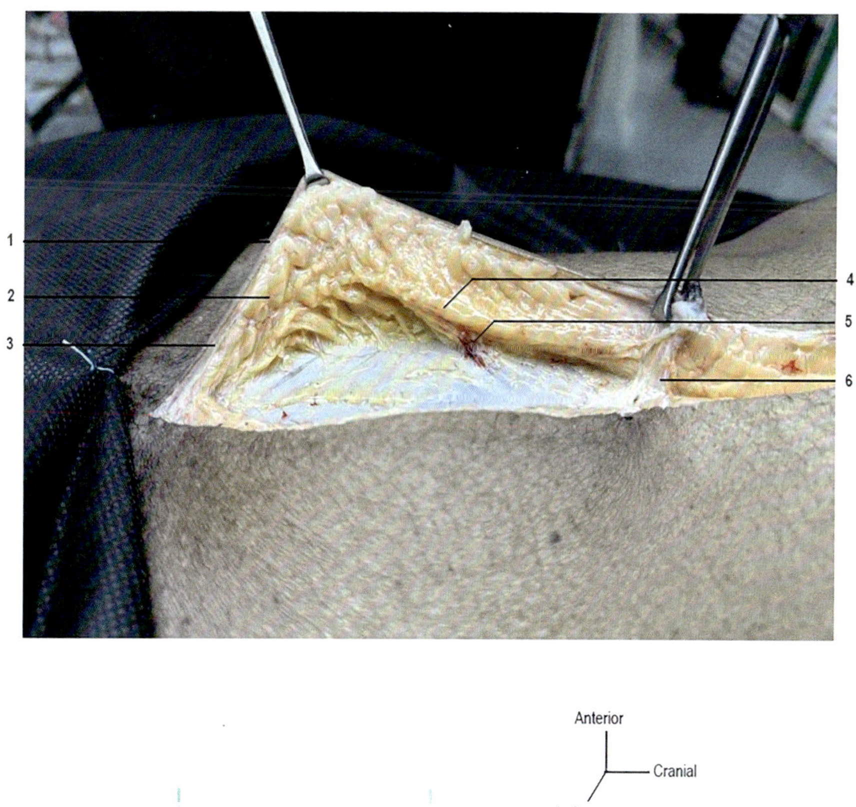

Fig. 5.2 Lateral view of subcutaneous tissue. (1) Epidermis; (2) Subcutaneous fat; (3) Dermis; (4) Fascia superficialis; (5) Perforating arteries; (6) Umbillicus insertion. (Credit: Dr. Paulo Barros)

The vertically oriented muscles include the rectus abdominis and the pyramidalis. The obliquely oriented muscles include the external oblique and the internal oblique. The horizontally oriented muscle corresponds to the transversus abdominis.

This variety of orientations provides the abdominal wall with strong resistance to deformation as well as significant mobility of the trunk.

5.2.2.1 Rectus Abdominis Muscle

Triangular in shape with a superior base, it inserts through three digitations on the external surface of ribs 5–7 and on the xiphoid process (Fig. 5.3). Its muscle body runs vertically downward. It is about 11 cm wide cranially, then narrows caudally to a tendon of 2–3 cm inserting on the superior part of the pubis and forming the Henle ligament [5].

It is divided by three to four tendinous intersections, which make it a polygastric muscle. These tendinous intersections are equivalent to lumbar vertebrae, similar to what is observed in reptiles. They reflect the metameric structure of the human body and give the muscle its characteristic appearance. Its distal insertion is on the superior surface of the pubis, between the pubic tubercle and the pubic angle.

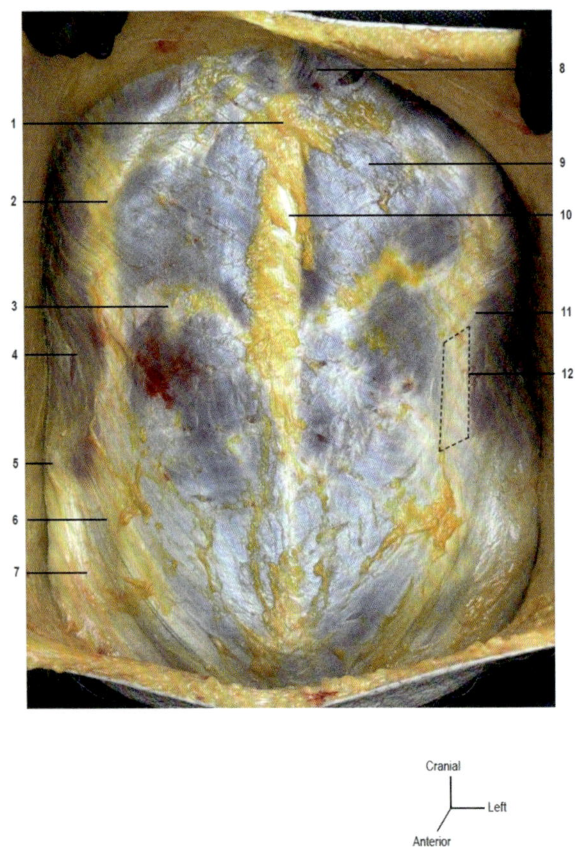

Fig. 5.3 Muscular first layer of the anterior abdominal wall. (1) Xiphoid process; (2) Costal margin, right tenth rib; (3) Tendinous intersection of the right rectus abdominis muscle; (4) Right external oblique muscle; (5) Anterior superior iliac spine; (6) Aponeurotic part of right external oblique muscle; (7) Inguinal ligament; (8) Proximal tendon of rectus abdominis muscle; (9) Left rectus abdominis muscle; (10) Linea alba; (11) Transition line between muscular and aponeurosis parts of left external oblique muscle; (12) Spigelian fascia. (Credit: Dr. Paulo Barros)

The rectus abdominis is surrounded by an aponeurosis formed by the union of the aponeuroses of the lateral muscles, called the rectus sheath. This sheath has two laminae, one anterior and one posterior. On the midline, the union of the right and left rectus sheaths forms the linea alba.

5.2.2.2 Pyramidalis Muscle

It is an inconstant muscle, present in 30% to 83% of individuals, depending on the series (Fig. 5.4) [6]. It originates from the pubis, runs upward and medially, and ends on the infraumbilical linea alba. A hypothetical role as a tensor of the linea alba has been suggested. However, it can also be considered as an accessory equivalent of the marsupial pouch [7, 8].

5.2.2.3 External Oblique Muscle

It is the most superficial of the three lateral muscles. It originates from the exothoracic surface of ribs 4–12, interdigitating with the fibers of the serratus anterior (ribs 5–9) and the latissimus dorsi (ribs 10–12) (Figs. 5.5, 5.6, and 5.7).

Its muscle body runs downward and forward, is relatively short, and ends in a long aponeurotic portion. Its aponeurosis contributes to the formation of the anterior lamina of the rectus sheath and the linea alba.

Inferiorly, it inserts on the iliac crest, the inguinal ligament, and the pubis, forming two crura. The lateral and medial crura form the superficial inguinal ring [9]. These crura are connected by intercrural fibers, described by Gillis and Nicaise, that close the superior part of the superficial inguinal ring.

5.2.2.4 Internal Oblique Muscle

Located beneath the external oblique, it represents the second layer of the lateral muscles (Figs. 5.6, 5.8, and 5.9). It originates from the thoracolumbar fascia and the anterior two-thirds of the iliac crest up to the anterior superior iliac spine.

Its fibers run upward and forward, perpendicular to the fibers of the external oblique. It ends medially in a wide aponeurotic portion. Cranially, this aponeurosis inserts on the chondro-costal margin of ribs 8–12.

More caudally, it contributes to the formation of the anterior and posterior laminae of the rectus sheath above the arcuate line. Below the arcuate line, its aponeurosis contributes only to the formation of the anterior lamina of the rectus sheath.

Inferiorly, its muscular fibers form an arch with the transversus abdominis around the spermatic cord in men and the round ligament in women, called the conjoint tendon. They insert distally on the lacunar ligament. At the inguinal level, some fibers contribute to the formation of the cremaster muscle.

5.2.2.5 Transverse Abdominis Muscle

Located beneath the internal oblique, it represents the third layer of the lateral muscles (Figs. 5.6, 5.9, and 5.10). Cranially, it inserts on the internal surface of ribs 7–10 and interdigitates with the fibers of the diaphragm on ribs 11 and 12.

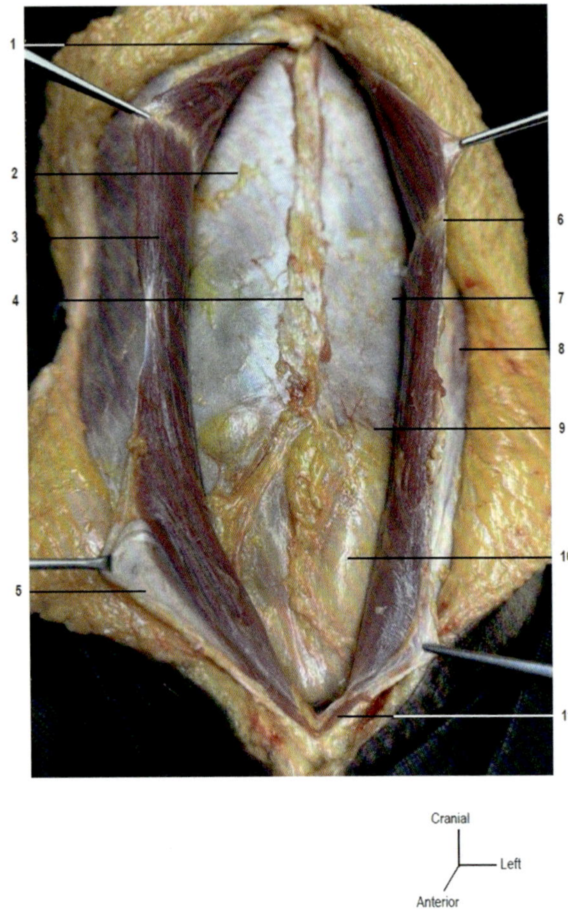

Fig. 5.4 Anterior view of retromuscular space. (1) Xiphoid process; (2) Right posterior rectus sheath; (3) Right rectus abdominis muscle; (4) Linea alba preserved after section of anterior rectus sheath; (5) Right anterior rectus sheath; (6) Tendinous intersection of the left rectus abdominis muscle; (7) Left posterior rectus sheath; (8) Left external oblique muscle; (9) Arcuate line of Douglas; (10) Preperitoneal space; (11) Sectioned pyramidalis muscle. (Credit: Dr. Paulo Barros)

Laterally and posteriorly, it attaches to the tips of the transverse processes of the lumbar vertebrae, the thoracolumbar fascia, the anterior half of the iliac crest, and the lateral third of the inguinal ligament. Its muscle body runs horizontally. Cranially, the muscle body of the transversus abdominis is very medial and may be seen during dissection of the retromuscular space.

It gives rise to a wide aponeurosis contributing to the posterior lamina of the rectus sheath above the arcuate line and to the anterior lamina below the arcuate line. At the inguinal level, its fibers merge with those of the internal oblique to form the conjoint tendon.

It plays a role in tightening the linea alba, supporting the abdominal organs, and expiration by pulling the ribs inward. The transversus abdominis muscle is also referred to as the "corset muscle" and is therefore considered the main antagonist of the diaphragm [10].

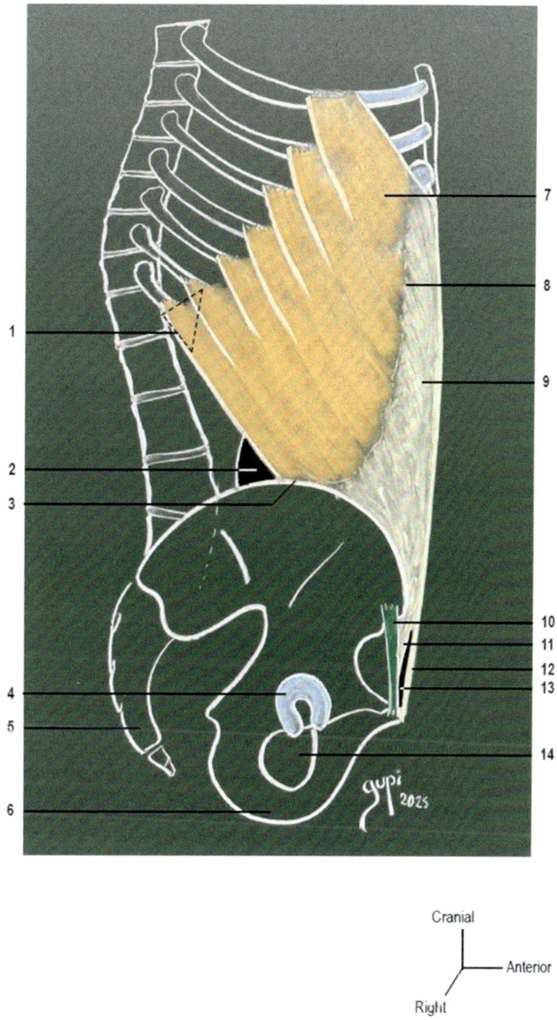

Fig. 5.5 External oblique muscle. (1) Superior lumbar triangle (Grynfeltt); (2) Inferior lumbar triangle (Petit); (3) Insertion half of the iliac crest; (4) Acetabulum; (5) Sacrum; (6) Ischium; (7) Muscular fibers covering the rectus abdominis muscle superiorly; (8) Transition line between muscular and aponeurosis parts; (9) Aponeurotic part forming the anterior rectus sheath; (10) Inguinal ligament; (11) Medial crura of the superficial inguinal ring; (12) Lateral crura of the superficial inguinal ring; (13) Superficial inguinal ring; (14) Obturator foramen

5.2.3 Aponeuroses and Transition Areas

5.2.3.1 Aponeurosis of the Lateral Muscles

The transition line of the external oblique muscle describes a posterior curve from the xiphoid process to the anterior superior iliac spine (Fig. 5.6). The transition line of the internal oblique muscle is also curved posteriorly in a concave manner. The transition line of the transversus abdominis muscle is sinuous from top to bottom and corresponds to the semilunar line. The line formed posterior to the rectus abdominis muscles by the anterior passage of the posterior lamina of the internal oblique aponeurosis and the transversus abdominis aponeurosis is called the arcuate line (of Douglas) [11, 12].

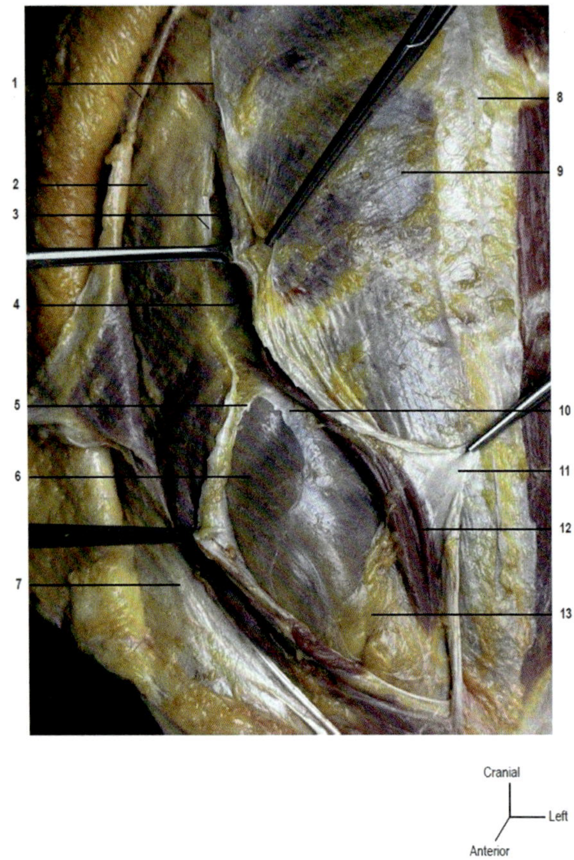

Fig. 5.6 Anterior view of lateral muscles' aponeuroses forming the rectus sheaths. (1) Sectioned external oblique muscle aponeurosis; (2) Right internal oblique muscle; (3) Sectioned internal oblique muscle aponeurosis; (4) Aponeurosis of transverse abdominis muscle; (5) Sectioned aponeurosis of transverse abdominis muscle (transverse abdominis release procedure); (6) Preperitoneal space; (7) Right inguinal ligament; (8) Linea alba; (9) Right rectus abdominis muscle. (Credit: Dr. Paulo Barros)

These transition zones are located at different levels. They should not be confused with the Spigelius line, which corresponds to the lateral border of the rectus abdominis. When it crosses the arcuate line of Douglas, it marks the location of the Spigelius point, the site of Spigelian hernias.

With the recent development of abdominal wall surgery and component separation techniques, some authors have proposed renaming the lateral border of the rectus abdominis as the "EIT Ambivium" and its intersection with the arcuate line of Douglas as the "Fulcrum abdominalis" [13].

5.2.3.2 Rectus Sheath

The rectus sheath is an aponeurotic sheath surrounding the rectus abdominis muscle (Fig. 5.4). It has two laminae, anterior and posterior, formed by the aponeuroses of the lateral muscles.

Above the arcuate line, located about 5 cm below the umbilicus, the external oblique forms the anterior lamina, the internal oblique contributes to both the

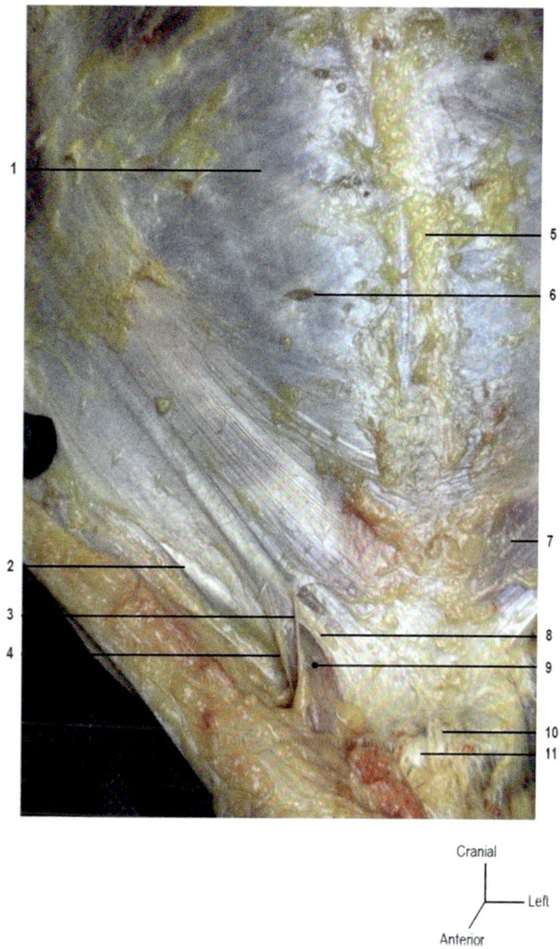

Fig. 5.7 Anterior view of external inguinal ring. (1) Right rectus abdominis muscle; (2) Inguinal ligament; (3) Right ilio-hypogastric nerve; (4) Lateral crura of the superficial inguinal ring; (5) Linea alba; (6) Perforating vessels orifice; (7) Left pyramidalis muscle; (8) Medial crura of the superficial inguinal ring; (9) Superficial inguinal ring; (10) Fundiform ligament of penis; (11) Pubis symphysis. (Credit: Dr. Paulo Barros)

anterior and posterior laminae, and the transversus abdominis forms the posterior lamina.

Below the arcuate line, the three lateral muscles contribute only to the anterior lamina, and there is no posterior lamina. This explains why an extended retromuscular dissection directed caudally enters the preperitoneal plane and can be continued into the inguinal region, as in the Stoppa procedure.

5.2.3.3 Linea Alba

The linea alba is an interlacing of aponeurotic fibers formed by the junction of the rectus sheaths on the midline (Fig. 5.3). It extends from the xiphoid process to the pubis, with a diamond-shaped anterior curvature and a maximal width at the umbilicus [14–16].

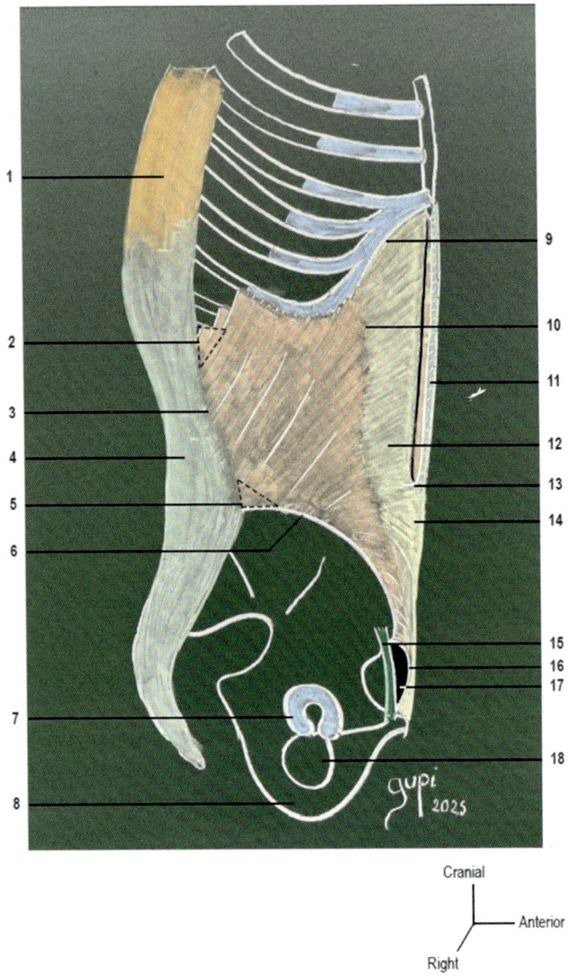

Fig. 5.8 Internal oblique muscle. (1) Latissimus dorsi muscle; (2) Superior lumbar triangle (Grynfeltt); (3) Posterior insertion on the thoraco-lumbar fascia; (4) Thoraco-lumbar fascia; (5) Inferior lumbar triangle (Petit); (6) Insertion anterior two-thirds of the iliac crest; (7) Acetabulum; (8) Ischium; (9) Superior insertion under the last ribs; (10) Transition line between the muscular and the aponeurosis parts; (11) Anterior lamina forming the anterior rectus sheath; (12) Posterior lamina forming the posterior rectus sheath; (13) Arcuate line of Douglas; (14) Anterior and posterior lamina passing anteriorly forming the anterior rectus sheath; (15) Inguinal ligament; (16) Falx inguinalis; (17) Deep inguinal ring; (18) Obturator foramen

Its width is variable and influenced by BMI, age, and sex. It is easy to identify above the umbilicus. Below the umbilicus, it may be so thin and covered by the pyramidalis muscle that it makes median laparotomy more difficult.

5.2.3.4 Umbilicus

The umbilicus is the fibrous scar of the former passage of the umbilical cord (Fig. 5.2). It forms a depression 2–8 mm wide, the depth of which depends on the adiposity of the subject. It is located slightly below the midpoint of the xiphopubic line and projected at the level of the L4 vertebra. It shows an external bulge on the surface and a circular groove in depth corresponding to the adhesion of the skin to the fibrous umbilical ring.

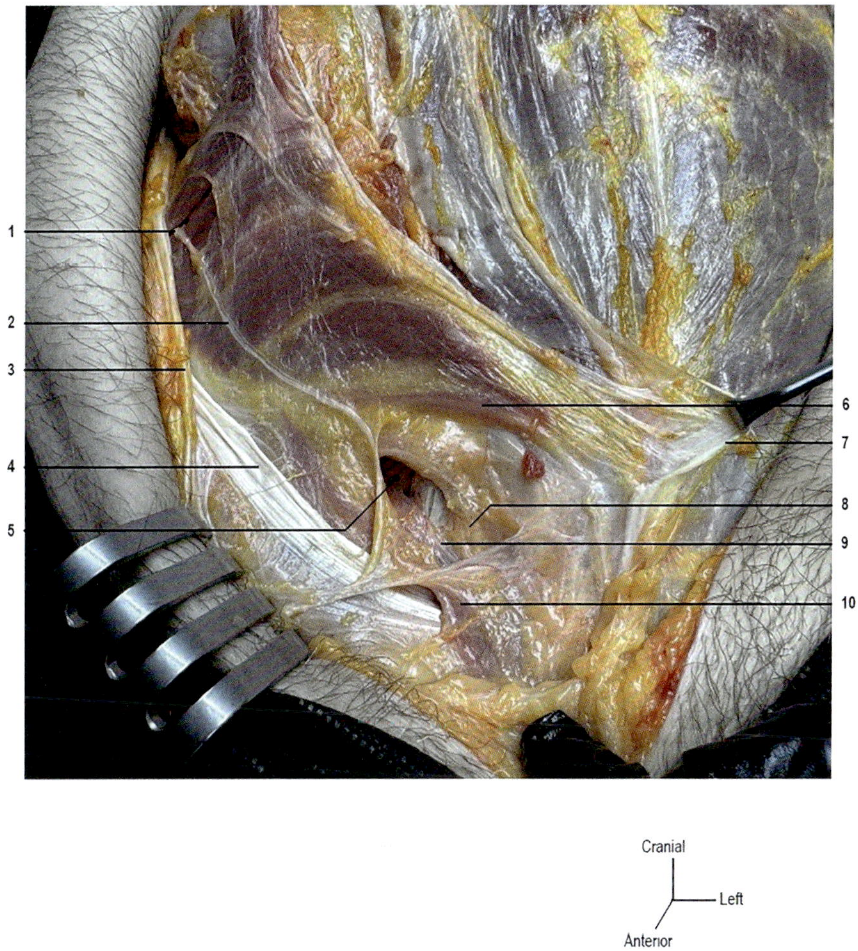

Fig. 5.9 Anterior view of internal inguinal ring. (1) Penetration of ilio-inguinal nerve between external oblique and internal oblique muscles; (2) Ilio-inguinal nerve; (3) Sectioned external oblique muscle aponeurosis; (4) Inguinal ligament; (5) Internal inguinal ring; (6) Falx inguinalis; (7) Sectioned external oblique muscle aponeurosis; (8) Fascia transversalis; (9) Genital branch of genito-femoral nerve; (10) Spermatic cord. (Credit: Dr. Paulo Barros)

Cranially, the round ligament of the liver, remnant of the left umbilical vein, inserts on the umbilicus. Caudally, a tripod is formed by the urachus (median umbilical ligament) and the remnants of the two umbilical arteries (medial umbilical ligaments). This natural weak zone of the abdominal wall is responsible for umbilical hernias, frequent in children and usually closing spontaneously with age.

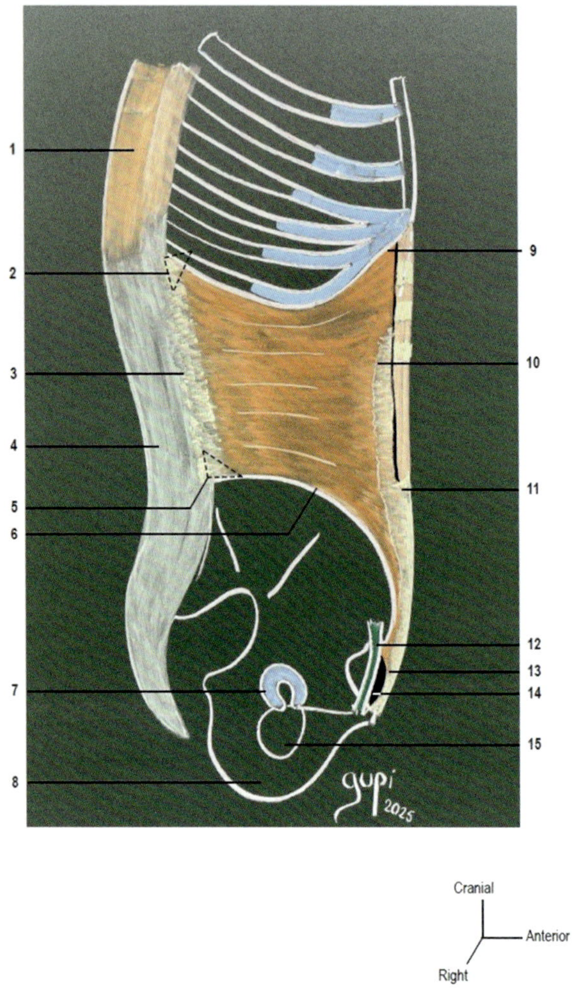

Fig. 5.10 Transverse abdominal muscle. (1) Latissimus dorsi muscle; (2) Superior lumbar triangle (Grynfeltt); (3) Posterior insertion on the thoraco-lumbar fascia with posterior aponeurosis; (4) Thoraco-lumbar fascia; (5) Inferior lumbar triangle (Petit); (6) Insertion anterior two-thirds of the iliac crest; (7) Acetabulum; (8) Ischium; (9) Superior insertion behind last ribs with diaphragm; (10) Transition line between muscular and aponeurosis parts = linea semilunaris; (11) Arcuate line of Douglas; (12) Inguinal ligament; (13) Falx inguinalis; (14) Deep inguinal ring; (15) Obturator foramen

5.2.4 Transversalis Fascia

It is a connective tissue layer covering the entire abdominal cavity [17]. Its thickness varies depending on location, and it takes different names accordingly, such as iliac fascia or psoas fascia.

This layer is thin when covering the transversus abdominis and becomes thicker caudally, forming the crural fascia, the interfoveolar ligament, and the iliopubic tract. It has been described with two layers, which are very difficult to distinguish during dissection of the anterior abdominal wall.

During preperitoneal dissection below the arcuate line, the correct plane is posterior to this fascia, in order to avoid injury to the epigastric vessels.

5.2.5 Preperitoneal Space

The preperitoneal space is a fatty areolar space located between the transversalis fascia and the peritoneum. Its thickness is variable and more developed beneath the linea alba and laterally toward the lumbar fossae.

It is continuous with the retroperitoneal space and with the preperitoneal pubic spaces of Retzius and Bogros. The space of Retzius lies between the pubis and the bladder. It is in this space that dissection is carried out to the pectineal ligament during transabdominal preperitoneal (TAPP) procedures.

The space of Bogros is continuous laterally with the space of Retzius up to the inguinal ligament. Dissection of this space is difficult laterally because of its thickness, requiring the surgeon to proceed carefully during a transversus abdominis release (TAR) procedure.

5.2.6 Parietal Peritoneum

As the deepest layer of the abdominal wall, it is almost adherent to the transversalis fascia at the level of the umbilicus and the diaphragm (Fig. 5.11). Along the midline, it is covered by preperitoneal fat, which provides an appropriate plane for prosthetic placement.

It shows four folds as it molds over the structures inserting on the umbilicus. Cranially, it covers the round ligament of the liver. Caudally and in the midline, it forms the median umbilical ligament by covering the urachus. Caudally and medially, it forms the medial umbilical ligaments and delineates the medial fossae. More laterally, it covers the epigastric pedicle, forming the lateral umbilical ligament and delineating the lateral fossae.

The supravesical fossa overlies the Hesselbach triangle, limited laterally by the Hesselbach ligament and cranially by the distal insertion of the rectus abdominis muscles.

5.3 Posterior Abdominal Wall (Lumbar Region)

It is the wall that closes the lumbar region posteriorly. Its general organization is similar to that of the anterior wall. The superficial planes (skin, subcutaneous tissue) and the deep planes (retroperitoneum, parietal peritoneum) will not be detailed here.

The musculo-aponeurotic wall can be divided into four layers.

5.3.1 First Layer

This is the most superficial muscular plane. It is composed of the latissimus dorsi, a large and wide muscle inserting on the thoracolumbar fascia, the spinous processes

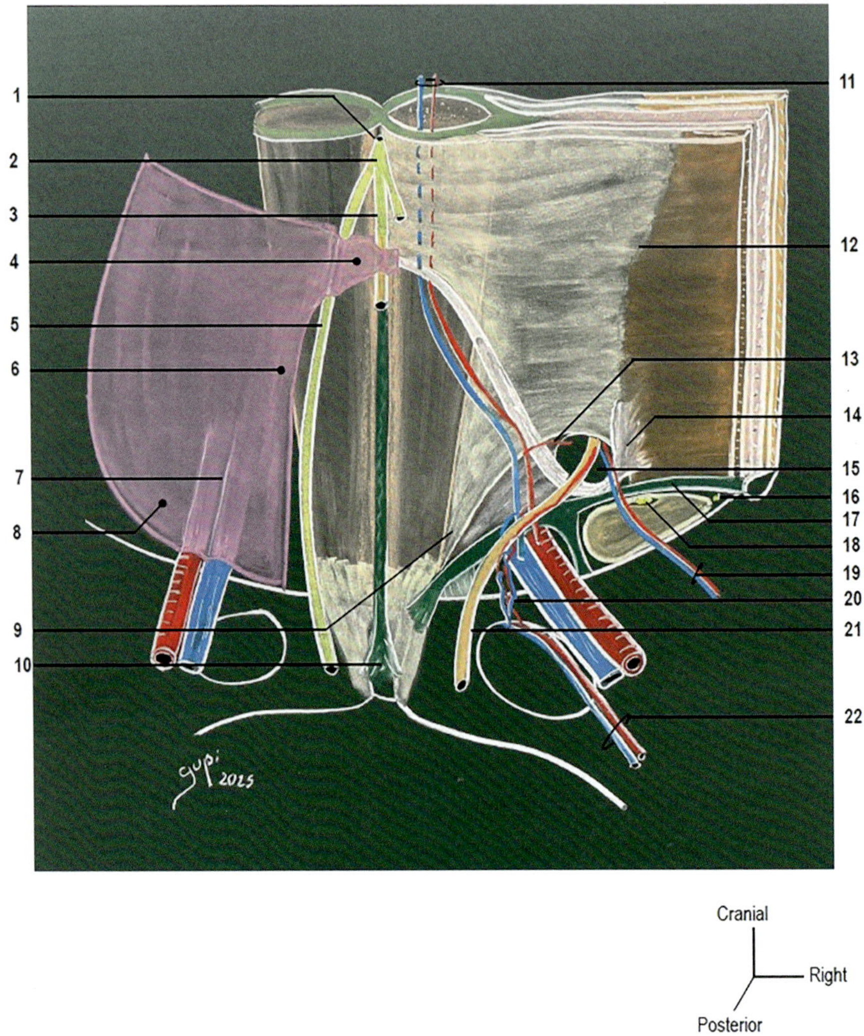

Fig. 5.11 Posterior view of inguinal region. (1) Round ligament of the liver; (2) Umbilicus; (3) Median umbilical ligament (obliterated urachus); (4) Supravesical fossae; (5) Lateral umbilical ligament (obliterated umbilical artery); (6) Medial umbilical fossae; (7) Lateral umbilical ligament (epigastric vessels); (8) Lateral umbilical fossae; (9) Hesselbach triangle; (10) Fundiform ligament of linea alba; (11) Epigastric vessels; (12) Transition line between muscular and aponeurosis parts = linea semilunaris; (13) Funicular artery; (14) Interfoveolar ligament of Hesselbach (part of transversalis fascia [TF]); (15) Deep inguinal ring with deep spermatic fascia (part of TF); (16) Lateral cutaneous nerve; (17) Inguinal ligament and ilio-pubic tract of Thompson (part of TF); (18) Femoral nerve; (19) Spermatic vessels; (20) Corona mortis vessels (anastomosis between the obturator and the external iliac or inferior epigastric vessels); (21) Vas deferent; (22) Obturator vessels

of T7 to L5, the median sacral crest, the iliac crest, ribs 8–12, the scapular angle, and the anterior surface of the humerus.

It covers the erector spinae muscles and partially the posterior part of the external oblique. At the superior part of the iliac crest, a lack of overlap with the external oblique defines the lumbar triangle (Jean Louis Petit), a weak area where lumbar hernias can occur.

5.3.2 Second Layer

Located beneath the latissimus dorsi, this layer includes the serratus posterior inferior and the internal oblique. The serratus posterior inferior overlaps the erector spinae muscles. It inserts on the thoracolumbar fascia, the spinous processes of T11 to L3, and ribs 8–12 by fleshy digitations on their inferior and posterior borders.

Together with the internal oblique, the inferior border of the 12th rib, and the superior edge of the iliac crest, it defines the lumbar quadrilateral (Grynfelt), another weak area where lumbar hernias may occur.

5.3.3 Third Layer

This deep layer is formed by the transversus abdominis and the costolumbar ligament. The costolumbar ligament extends from the transverse processes of L1 and L2 to ribs 11 and 12.

5.3.4 Fourth Layer

This is the deepest plane of the posterior wall. It is formed by the quadratus lumborum, located anterior to the aponeurosis of the transversus abdominis. It is a quadrilateral muscle inserting superiorly on the inferior border of the 12th rib and inferiorly on the iliac crest. Medially, it attaches to the transverse processes of the lumbar vertebrae.

In surgery, it is rarely directly visualized. It represents the posterior limit of preperitoneal dissection during neurectomy through a posterior approach.

5.4 Vascularization

5.4.1 Arterial Supply

The arterial supply of the abdominal wall is organized into a superficial subcutaneous network and a deep musculo-aponeurotic network. These two networks are widely anastomosed. The deep network includes a vertical system and a transversal system, which will be described separately.

5.4.1.1 Deep Network/Vertical System

The vertical system arises from the inferior epigastric artery on each side. This artery originates from the external iliac artery, medial to the deep inguinal ring, which it bypasses along its medial border. At its origin, it creates a fold on the peritoneum called the lateral umbilical ligament, which must be considered during peritoneal incision in TAPP procedures.

Its course runs cranially, following the interfoveolar ligament of Hesselbach, then crosses posterior to the rectus abdominis about 4–8 cm above the pubis. At this level, it runs along the posterior surface of the rectus abdominis, above the transversalis fascia. Care is required during retromuscular dissection below the arcuate line, where dissection above the transversalis fascia may injure the epigastric vessels.

It gives off two branches: an inferior branch that anastomoses with the obturator artery, and a superior branch that anastomoses with the superior epigastric artery from the internal thoracic artery. A full-channel anastomosis between the superior and inferior epigastric systems occurs in about 20% of cases. In most situations, this connection corresponds to a network of collateral branches from the two distinct arteries.

5.4.1.2 Deep Network/Transversal System

The transversal system reflects the segmental arrangement of the human body. It is represented mainly by the last six intercostal arteries, the subcostal arteries, and the lumbar arteries, which course between the internal oblique and the transversus abdominis.

This system is reinforced cranially by the musculophrenic artery and caudally by the deep circumflex iliac artery, a branch of the external iliac artery, which runs on the deep surface of the inguinal ligament. These vessels anastomose with the vertical system after crossing the posterior lamina of the rectus sheath.

Care must be taken during retromuscular dissection, where extending dissection too laterally may injure these arteries. They may also be injured during drain insertion into the flanks.

5.4.1.3 Superficial Network

The superficial arterial network consists of perforating arteries that supply the subcutaneous tissue and the skin [18]. W.E. Huger described three zones to explain the superficial blood supply of the abdomen [19].

Zone I refers to the superior and central abdomen. Zone II refers to the inferior abdomen. Zone III refers to the superior and lateral abdomen. Cutaneous branches of Zone I originate from the deep superior epigastric artery. Cutaneous branches of Zone III come from the deep lateral-transversal system. Cutaneous branches of Zone II come from the deep lateral-transversal system, the inferior epigastric artery, and the superficial circumflex iliac artery, the latter arising from the femoral artery.

At the level of the umbilicus, four perforating arteries form a well-developed peri-umbilical anastomotic circle.

5.4.2 Venous Supply

The venous network parallels the arterial one and can be highly complex. The superior network drains into the superior vena cava, while the inferior network drains into the inferior vena cava, thus creating a cava-caval anastomosis. This network also communicates with the venous system of the round ligament at the umbilicus, forming a porto-caval anastomosis, which may recanalize in cirrhotic patients.

5.4.3 Lymphatic Drainage

The lymphatic system includes a superficial and a deep network.

The superficial network is highly diffuse. It drains caudally toward the inguinal and lumbar regions and cranially toward the intercostal and internal thoracic lymphatic systems. Laterally, it forms a chain of lymph nodes along the mammary line.

The deep network drains cranially toward the internal thoracic chain, laterally toward the lumbar nodes, and caudally toward the external iliac chain and the inguinal nodes. The umbilicus provides a connection with the deep hepatic and pelvic lymphatic networks.

5.5 Innervation

Motor, sensory, nociceptive, and proprioceptive innervation arises from intercostal nerves T7 to T12 and from lumbar roots L1 and L2, which give rise to the ilioinguinal, iliohypogastric, and genitofemoral nerves. These nerves run between the transversus abdominis and the internal oblique before entering the posterior rectus sheath [20].

This plane, called the transversus abdominis plane (TAP), is the target of TAP blocks, a technique of regional anesthesia for the abdominal wall. During retromuscular dissection, the surgeon must avoid excessive lateral dissection, which may injure the neurovascular bundles and denervate the rectus abdominis. Dissection should remain close to the posterior rectus sheath, leaving the nerves and vessels in contact with the rectus muscle.

The nerves arising from L1 and L2 pass between the internal oblique and the external oblique at the groin. At this level, regional anesthesia is referred to as ilioinguinal block or iliohypogastric block.

The skin follows a metameric innervation pattern through perforating branches. These perforators may be the source of highly localized pain, as seen in syndromes such as Cyriax, Tietze, and Maigne [20].

5.6 Conclusion

The abdominal wall surgeon must have a precise knowledge of parietal anatomy before considering any repair.

Understanding muscular anatomy allows safe dissection through the different planes. It ensures effective placement of prosthetic material and properly performed component separations. Knowledge of vascular and nerve anatomy helps to avoid severe complications such as hematomas or denervation, both of which are risk factors for recurrence.

Mastering the dissection of these planes makes it possible to plan complex repairs of multiple ventral hernias, whether lateral, medial, or inguinal.

References

1. Flament JB. Functional anatomy of the abdominal wall. Chirurg. 2006;77(5):401–7.
2. Caix M, Cubertafond P. Etude anatomique de la région thoraco-abdominale considérée en fonction du type morphologique. Anat Clin. 1978;1:185–8.
3. On the anatomy and physiology of the skin. I. The cleavability of the cutis. (Translated from Langer, K. (1861). Zur Anatomie und Physiologie der Haut. I. Uber die Spaltbarkeit der Cutis. Sitzungsbericht der Mathematisch-naturwissenschaftlichen Classe der Kaiserlichen Academie der Wissenschaften, 44, 19.). Br J Plast Surg. 1978;31(1):3–8.
4. Lemperle G, Tenenhaus M, Knapp D, Lemperle SM. The direction of optimal skin incisions derived from striae distensae. Plast Reconstr Surg. 2014;134(6):1424–34.
5. Gnanadev R, Iwanaga J, Oskouian RJ, et al. Henle's ligament: a comprehensive review of its anatomy and terminology over almost one and a half centuries. Cureus. 2018;10(9):e3366.
6. Hojaij FC, Kogima RO, Moyses RA, et al. Morphometry and frequency of the pyramidalis muscle in adult humans: a pyramidalis muscle's anatomical analysis. Clinics. 2020;75:e1623.
7. Cirocchi R, Cheruiyot I, Henry BM, et al. Anatomical variations of the pyramidalis muscle: a systematic review and meta-analysis. Surg Radiol Anat. 2021;43(4):595–605.
8. Das SS, Saluja S, Vasudeva N. Biometrics of pyramidalis muscle and its clinical importance. J Clin Diagn Res. 2017;11(2):AC05-7.
9. Baqué P, Hekayem L. Leçons d'anatomie. 1st ed. Paris: Ellipses; 2022.
10. Urquhart DM, Barker PJ, Hodges PW, et al. Regional morphology of the transversus abdominis and obliquus internus and externus abdominis muscles. Clin Biomech. 2005;20(3):233–41.
11. Loukas M, Myers C, Shah R, et al. Arcuate line of the rectus sheath: clinical approach. Anat Sci Int. 2008;83(3):140–4.
12. Montgomery A, Petersson U, Austrums E. The arcuate line hernia: operative treatment and a review of the literature. Hernia. 2013;17(3):391–6.
13. Vierstraete M, Pereira Rodriguez JA, Renard Y, Muysoms F. EIT ambivium, linea semilunaris, and fulcrum abdominalis. J Abdom Wall Surg. 2023;2:12217.
14. Mota P, Pascoal AG, Carita AI, Bø K. The immediate effects on inter-rectus distance of abdominal crunch and drawing-in exercises during pregnancy and the postpartum period. J Orthop Sports Phys Ther. 2015;45(10):781–8.
15. Rath AM, Attali P, Dumas JL, et al. The abdominal linea alba: an anatomo-radiologic and biomechanical study. Surg Radiol Anat. 1996;18(4):281–8.
16. Gueroult P, Joppin V, Chaumoitre K, et al. Linea alba 3D morphometric variability by CT scan exploration. Hernia. 2024;28(2):485–94.

17. Peiper C, Junge K, Prescher A, et al. Abdominal musculature and the transversalis fascia: an anatomical viewpoint. Hernia. 2004;8(4):376–80.
18. Gandhi J, Banker A, Chaudhari S, Shinde P. Role of indocyanine green to mitigate wound complications in component separation technique for ventral hernia repair—our early experience. World J Surg. 2021;45(10):3073–9.
19. Huger WE Jr. The anatomic rationale for abdominal lipectomy. Am Surg. 1979;45(9):612–7.
20. Anatomie des nerfs craniens et rachidiens et du système grand sympathique, chez l'homme. Arch NeurPsych. 1927;18(1):154–5.

Part II

Surgical Techniques and Strategies

Management of Large Incisional Hernias

6

Niccolò Grappolini, Marta Cavalli, Piero Bruni,
Livia Manfredini, and Giampiero Campanelli

6.1 Definition of "Large Incisional Hernia"

According to the classification proposed by the European Hernia Society (EHS), a "large incisional hernia" is characterized by a defect measuring at least 10 cm in width along the midline (defined as W3). When this is combined with the concept of loss of domain, the hernia is classified as a "giant ventral hernia" or "abdominal wall disaster". Ventral hernias are considered massive when they exhibit a width or length of at least 15 cm or an overall defect area exceeding 150 cm^2 [1]. Loss of domain is a key concept in the assessment of complex hernias. It is defined as a condition in which more than 20% of the visceral contents are chronically located outside the abdominal cavity. This scenario leads to altered abdominal-thoracic pressure dynamics and significantly complicates the reintegration of herniated contents into the intra-abdominal space. Consequently, there is an increased risk of postoperative abdominal compartment syndrome, respiratory compromise, and visceral ischemia. Preoperative evaluation of this condition can be performed using volumetric computed tomography (CT) imaging, with the calculation of various indices, including the "Love", "Sabbagh", and "Tanaka" indices, which will be discussed in detail later [2]. A main aspect in defining a giant hernia is the functional impairment of the abdominal wall. Large incisional hernias often result in chronic alterations of abdominal wall biomechanics, including loss of muscle tone, atrophy, fibrosis, retraction of the rectus and oblique muscles, and alteration of the abdominal-pelvic pressure equilibrium. These changes manifest clinically with both systemic and local symptoms such as chronic pain, incontinence, walking disorders, and functional limitations. In such cases, surgery is not only structural repair but also assumes a reconstructive and rehabilitative role [3, 4].

N. Grappolini · M. Cavalli · P. Bruni · L. Manfredini · G. Campanelli (✉)
IRCCS Ospedale Galeazzi – Sant'Ambrogio (Hernia Center Milano), University of Insubria, Milan, Italy
e-mail: giampiero.campanelli@grupposandonato.it

D. Cuccurullo, C. Rispoli (eds.), *Complex Abdominal Wall Surgery*, Updates in Surgery, https://doi.org/10.1007/978-3-032-24284-6_6

6.2 Prehabilitation

The concept of prehabilitation in the management of complex hernias represents one of the most significant advancements in recent surgical practice. This approach is based on the idea that preoperative patient optimization, through targeted strategies aimed at risk reduction and anatomical enhancement, can improve surgical outcomes and reduce complications.

In the repair of complex abdominal wall hernias, prehabilitation techniques primarily aim to facilitate the reintegration of visceral contents into the abdominal cavity, increase abdominal wall compliance, and reduce the risk of complications and compartment syndrome. Accurate anatomical assessment of the defect, typically through dynamic CT imaging, along with a thorough evaluation of the patient's overall condition, constitutes an essential first step [3]. One of the most established tools in this setting is preoperative progressive pneumoperitoneum (PPP), first introduced by Goñi Moreno in the 1940s and recently revisited seeing the growing incidence of hernias with loss of domain [5]. The principle behind PPP involves the gradual insufflation of air into the peritoneal cavity through a catheter placed under ultrasound or CT guidance. Insufflations are performed daily or on alternate days over a period of 7–14 days, achieving total volumes of 2000–4000 mL. PPP promotes abdominal wall adaptation, increases compliance, and enlarges intra-abdominal volume (25–40%), improving visceral repositioning tolerance. The risks include pneumothorax, pneumomediastinum, subcutaneous emphysema, gas embolism, and, rarely, bowel perforation. For this reason, PPP should be performed in specialized centers with appropriate radiologic and clinical monitoring. It is contraindicated in patients with severe COPD, recent thromboembolic events, or uncontrolled coagulopathies [6]. As an alternative or in conjunction with PPP, preoperative botulinum toxin type A (BTX-A) injection into the abdominal wall has gained traction as a safe and less invasive technique. Its physiological rationale lies in the temporary flaccid paralysis induced in the oblique and transversus abdominis muscles, resulting in muscle relaxation and elongation. This effect, achieved through ultrasound-guided bilateral injections, allows for medial advancement of the fascial edge (often exceeding 5 cm per side) facilitating tension-free closure of the defect. BTX-A is typically injected at 5–6 sites per side, with a total dose ranging from 200 to 300 units distributed among the three muscles. The effect becomes apparent within 5–7 days and lasts for approximately 2–3 months, providing a favorable window for surgical intervention under optimal anatomical conditions. Multiple studies have demonstrated a significant reduction in the need for component separation, suture line tension, and postoperative complications in patients receiving preoperative BTX-A [7–9]. Proper patient selection is crucial to the effectiveness of these techniques. The Tanaka score is a valuable tool based on the ratio between the volume of herniated contents and the total abdominal cavity volume, calculated via three-dimensional CT imaging. A ratio greater than 20% (Tanaka index >0.2) typically indicates loss of domain and supports the indication for prehabilitation strategies. Ratios exceeding 30–35% are associated with a high risk of primary closure failure and postoperative compartment syndrome, making the use of PPP and BTX-A nearly indispensable [10]. Alternative scoring systems include the Sabbagh index (2011) [11], which considers a ratio between hernia and peritoneal volume below 20% as predictive of tension-free fascial closure, and the Love index (2021) [12], which evaluates the width of the rectus muscles relative to the width of the defect. This ratio, termed the Rectus Defect Ratio (RDR), if greater than two, is associated with up to 90% probability of achieving tension-free fascial closure. Lastly, but not least, to facilitate the patient's optimal condition upon arrival in the operating room, a structured respiratory and nutritional prehabilitation will be essential. On the respiratory side, a tailored program including incentive spirometry, inspiratory muscle training, and respiratory physiotherapy is recommended to enhance thoraco-pulmonary compliance and prevent postoperative complications such as atelectasis or respiratory failure. Simultaneously, nutritional optimization involves a patient-specific approach: a hypocaloric, normoproteic diet for obese individuals; a high-protein diet in cases of sarcopenia or muscular deficiency; and a low-residue (low-fiber) diet in the days preceding surgery to minimize intestinal volume and facilitate fascial closure [3, 4].

6.3 The Role of Obesity

Obesity is one of the principal modifiable risk factors in the pathogenesis, progression, and recurrence of large incisional hernias and must be considered as part of prehabilitation. Numerous clinical studies have demonstrated a direct correlation between elevated BMI and increased risk of hernia recurrence, surgical site infection, seroma formation, wound dehiscence, and respiratory complications. From a pathophysiological standpoint, obesity profoundly alters the biomechanics of the abdominal wall. Excess visceral and subcutaneous adipose tissue contributes to a chronically elevated intra-abdominal pressure, leading to fascial distension, progressive stretching of the rectus and oblique muscles, and a loss of structural integrity of the abdominal wall. Additionally, fatty infiltration within the abdominal muscles reduces contractile strength and endurance, resulting in abdominal wall dysfunction that impairs postoperative healing. Beyond biomechanical effects, obesity induces systemic alterations that negatively affect wound healing. Impaired immune responses, reduced local hygiene due to body habitus, and increased mechanical stress on surgical closures contribute to the high incidence of local complications observed in obese patients [13]. Obesity also poses significant technical challenges. The thick adipose pannus hampers access to anatomical planes, complicates the identification of fascial margins, and increases the risk of iatrogenic injuries. Furthermore, mesh positioning, fixation, and tissue integration are more technically demanding, with higher risks of mesh displacement and migration [14]. Given these considerations, preoperative weight optimization is an essential step in the management of obese patients with complex hernias. Major surgical guidelines recommend preoperative weight loss through a multidisciplinary approach involving dietitians, physiotherapists, psychologists, and, in selected cases, bariatric surgeons. The American Hernia Society and the World Society of Abdominal Compartment Syndrome consider a BMI >40 a relative contraindication to elective complex hernia repair. In such scenarios, a stepwise approach is preferred: initial bariatric surgery, followed by a period of nutritional and functional stabilization and, finally, abdominal wall reconstruction, possibly combined with prehabilitation techniques. This has been our strategy for decades [15]. In selected cases, combined bariatric and hernia surgery may represent a viable option, but it should be reserved for high-volume centers with established multidisciplinary expertise. Regardless of the surgical strategy, appropriate patient selection, optimization of metabolic and respiratory comorbidities, and adequate nutritional and physical prehabilitation are essential prerequisites to reduce perioperative risk and improve long-term outcomes [16].

6.4 Indications: Open Surgery Versus Minimally Invasive Surgery

The surgical management of large incisional hernias requires a tailored approach based on multiple factors, including the characteristics of the defect, the patient's clinical condition, and the expertise of the multidisciplinary team. Historically, the open approach has represented the gold standard for the treatment of large incisional hernias, especially in cases with significant loss of domain, multiple or "Swiss cheese" defects, complex recurrences, and clinical scenarios involving marked anatomical and functional compromise. This approach allows for direct and complete exposure of the defect, extensive mobilization of fascial flaps and, when necessary, resection of scar tissue, fistulas, or infected mesh. In cases properly classified as large incisional hernias, as mentioned above, this remains our preferred approach. The use of prosthetic materials (synthetic, biologic, or biosynthetic) has become mandatory to significantly reduce recurrence rates. The reference technique is the Rives-Stoppa repair, which involves retrorectus preperitoneal mesh placement extending from the xiphoid process to the pubis (cranio-caudally) and laterally to the semilunar lines. In all the new techniques of component separation available today, the possibility to extend in this surgical plane is essential in the case of large incisional hernias [3]. On the other hand, technological advancements and increasing expertise in laparoscopic and robotic techniques have led some surgical teams to extend minimally invasive indications to medium and large hernias in selected patients. Since the early 1990s, laparoscopic intraperitoneal onlay mesh (IPOM) techniques gained popularity for the repair of large hernias—a strategy we no longer endorse. More recently, thanks to the introduction of new techniques such as the transabdominal preperitoneal (TAPP) technique, which places the mesh in the preperitoneal space, and the extended-view totally extraperitoneal (e-TEP) approach, we have expanded the scope of extraperitoneal repair for larger defects. These approaches allow for retrorectus mesh positioning with improved tissue integration and reduced long-term complications. While IPOM has been widely used for small to medium defects, it poses limitations in complex hernias, particularly due to the risk of visceral adhesions and challenges in managing loss of domain. Additionally, postoperative pain is often greater due to the use of tacks on the posterior fascia. The e-TEP approach, although valuable, has limitations in terms of initial access, peritoneal dissection, especially in obese patients or those with adhesions. The introduction of the robotic approach has totally revolutionized the field. The possibility to reach easily the retrorectus-preperitoneal space, the simplicity of performing lateral isolation and the user-friendly suture systems have led many surgeons (including ourselves) to gradually adopt the minimally invasive procedure from simple ventral hernia to complex incisional hernia. Laparoscopic TAPP is technically demanding, but robotic TAPP (r-TAPP) combines the advantages of ideal mesh placement—with coverage comparable to open surgery—and minimally invasive access, enhanced by 3D visualization and articulated instrumentation. In our experience, r-TAPP now represents a valid option for medium-to-large defects and can be considered the gold standard among minimally invasive techniques, as well as for primary ventral hernias plus diastasis from small to medium dimension. Nonetheless, it does not replace open surgery, particularly in complex or catastrophic abdominal wall situations. Robotic surgery, in particular, has shown promising results in the repair of complex hernias, enabling precise dissection, advanced intracorporeal suturing, and even posterior component separation in a minimally invasive environment. Techniques such as robotic transversus abdominis release (r-TAR) allow for wide muscular mobilization with low morbidity, while preserving the benefits of minimal invasiveness [17, 18].

6.5 Component Separation Techniques

Component separation techniques are reconstructive surgical approaches used to achieve tension-free closure of large abdominal wall defects by mobilizing and advancing the rectus muscles medially, expanding the available surface area for mesh placement. Initially described by Ramirez in 1990, this strategy revolutionized abdominal wall reconstruction [19]. Anterior component separation (ACS)—known as the Ramirez technique—was originally developed to enable closure of large midline defects without the use of prosthetic mesh. However, contemporary practice typically includes mesh placement to reinforce the repair and reduce recurrence rates. The critical step in ACS involves extensive bilateral subcutaneous dissection extending caudally to the inguinal ligament, cranially beyond the costal margin, and laterally 2–3 cm past the semilunar line to expose the external oblique aponeurosis. A longitudinal incision 1–2 cm lateral to the semilunar line releases the external oblique, permitting medial advancement of the muscle-fascial complex. The rectus abdominis and conjoined internal oblique/transversus abdominis aponeuroses are thus freed from lateral tethering, enabling central closure. Classical cadaveric studies have demonstrated that ACS permits medial advancement of up to

10 cm in the epigastric region, 20 cm at the umbilicus, and 6–8 cm in the suprapubic area per side, sufficient for the closure of defects up to ~20 cm in width. An additional advantage is that the advanced muscular flaps remain innervated and vascularized, offering better functional outcomes than free flap transfers, which tend to result in muscle atrophy over time. Nonetheless, anterior separation has notable disadvantages. The most significant is that the dissection compromises midline skin vascularization by disrupting perforating vessels, especially problematic in obese or smoking patients. This increases the risk of wound complications such as seroma, hematoma, surgical site infection, wound dehiscence, and even partial skin necrosis. Postoperative pain is also a relevant concern: ACS is a relatively extensive and disruptive procedure. Incision of the external oblique disrupts lateral musculoaponeurotic continuity and, if not repaired appropriately, may predispose to lateral bulging or secondary hernias. Hernia recurrence is another consideration, with medium-term rates of 10–20% for ACS without mesh. Some patients may experience chronic discomfort or abdominal paresthesia due to transection of small cutaneous nerve branches [20]. As for the endoscopic anterior component separation (EACS), introduced and described in 2007 by Jorgensen and Jensen, this is commonly used in combination with retromuscular mesh placement according to the Rives-Stoppa technique. The approach involves access to the plane between the external and internal oblique muscles through a small lateral incision, expansion of the space with a balloon, and then controlled incision of the external oblique aponeurosis. This allows for sufficient myofascial release to achieve tension-free midline closure. The main advantages of EACS include a very low infection rate (less than 1% in the dissection area), a reduced incidence of seromas (around 5%, usually self-limiting), and the possibility to avoid the use of bridged mesh, even in patients with defects larger than 20 cm [21]. In the past, about 25 years ago, we reported a pioneering experience with the use of a double mesh technique for large incisional hernias with loss of abdominal wall substance: an absorbable mesh (Vicryl™) to reconstruct the peritoneal plane and a non-absorbable mesh (Marlex™) in the retromuscular position for long-term reinforcement. At the time, it was an innovative approach designed to reduce complications from direct mesh-bowel contact and to restore abdominal wall anatomy without tension when the component separation is not enough. The results showed low mortality, few serious complications, and no recurrences [3, 22]. Today, this concept is widely accepted. Posterior component separation with transversus abdominis release (TAR) is a more recent technical evolution designed to manage complex ventral hernias [23]. TAR is particularly indicated for large incisional hernias (fascial defect width >10 cm), loss of domain, or defects in anatomically challenging locations such as lateral, lumbar, or subcostal regions. It allows placement of large meshes with wide overlap. The key maneuver in TAR is the release of the transversus abdominis muscle, which is incised medially along its aponeurotic insertion on the posterior rectus sheath. This dissection separates the transversus muscle and aponeurosis from the underlying transversalis fascia. Importantly, the segmental intercostal nerves (which run between the internal oblique and transversus to innervate the rectus) are preserved, as the incision is

medial to their entry points into the musculature. Once released, the transversus muscle retracts, no longer resisting medialization of the posterior sheath. Mesh is then placed in a retromuscular, extraperitoneal, retrotransversus plane with oblique muscles intact and the rectus innervated. Recently we proposed a real and innovative alternative that introduced a new surgical approach for abdominal wall reconstruction: anterior compartment mobilization (ACM) through a posterior approach. It allows the mobilization of the anterior compartment, made by the rectus muscle and its anterior sheath and the posterior compartment that includes the posterior sheath of the rectus muscle, the transversalis fascia, and the peritoneum. The key innovation is that ACM can be combined with TAR in the same procedure when both the anterior and posterior compartments are damaged, in cases of parietal disaster and real loss of substance of both compartments. This dual approach enables tension-free midline closure and a very large mesh placement while ensuring the functional integrity of the abdominal wall [24]. However, TAR also presents limitations and requires careful consideration. It is anatomically complex and demands a thorough understanding of deep fascial planes, as well as advanced retromuscular dissection skills. The learning curve is steep, and technical errors can lead to specific complications: for instance, overly lateral incisions of the transversus muscle may damage intercostal nerves, and incomplete closure of the posterior sheath may result in interparietal herniation—the so-called "Mickey Mouse hernias"—where herniated viscera protrude around the mesh, producing a characteristic radiologic appearance [25]. Another drawback is that in the event of deep infection or wound dehiscence, the mesh lies in a deeper anatomical plane and may become involved. Seroma formation, although less frequent than with ACS, can still occur. In conclusion, the choice between anterior and posterior component separation depends on the clinical context and the need for advancement of the anterior or posterior compartment. TAR has increasingly gained popularity for the treatment of complex incisional hernias due to its technical advantages and reduced wound morbidity, but it requires specific expertise. The implementation of these techniques has enabled successful repair of previously inoperable defects, improving both functional and aesthetic outcomes for patients [26, 27].

6.6 The Meshes

Biosynthetic meshes represent a significant advancement in abdominal wall reconstruction, particularly in the treatment of large incisional hernias in high-risk settings—such as contaminated fields or compromised tissue quality or in the case of real loss of substance of posterior compartment where they can be easily used to replace it. These materials were developed to bridge the gap between permanent synthetic meshes and biologic matrices, offering the mechanical strength of traditional synthetic meshes with enhanced biocompatibility and a physiological remodeling process that more closely mimics native tissue behavior. However, four synthetic materials frequently used in the repair of large incisional hernias, even in high-risk settings, deserve special mention. The two most common, polypropylene and polyester, are characterized by excellent tissue integration and handling but are associated with a high risk of adhesions when in direct contact with the viscera. Polyester, in particular, is less suitable in cases of highly potential contaminated surgical field. In addition, two other materials are increasingly employed thanks to several advantages: polyvinylidene fluoride (PVDF) and polytetrafluoroethylene (PTFE). Both belong to the class of fluoropolymers, known for their high chemical and biological inertness and non-absorbability, but they are very different in structure, tissue interaction, and clinical indications. PVDF is typically configured in wide-pore meshes (~2 mm), promoting solid tissue integration and a more controlled and stable inflammatory response over time. In contrast, PTFE, particularly in its expanded form (e-PTFE), is a microporous mesh (<10 μm) offering a highly flexible and inert profile. This makes it preferable in intraperitoneal repairs, as it significantly reduces the risk of visceral adhesions. However, its limited porosity increases the risk of seroma, chronic infection, and capsular fibrosis [28, 29]. Unlike permanent meshes, biosynthetic meshes are composed of resorbable polymers designed to maintain sufficient tensile strength for a defined period (typically 3–6 months) while promoting cellular infiltration, neovascularization, and tissue remodeling. The main categories include fully synthetic resorbable polymers and biologically derived matrices from decellularized porcine or bovine collagen, processed to reduce immunogenicity. Among the most widely studied biosynthetic meshes are Phasix™ (P4HB), Synecor™ (PTFE + PGA:TMC), and TIGR® Matrix (a dual-phase copolymer), each offering distinct profiles regarding degradation kinetics, inflammatory response, and residual mechanical strength. The primary indication for biosynthetic mesh use is the repair of complex hernias in contaminated or potentially contaminated fields, such as in the presence of enterocutaneous fistulas, ostomies, or previous mesh infections, especially in frail or immunocompromised patients. In these scenarios, available evidence suggests that biosynthetic meshes may reduce the incidence of severe infectious complications and reoperation rates while maintaining satisfactory short- to mid-term durability. Biosynthetics can also be used to reconstruct the posterior layer in combination with a permanent synthetic mesh used for the primary repair, as stated above [22]. Since both biologic and synthetic substrate materials each have a unique set of advantages and drawbacks, hybrid meshes were recently developed, such as biologic decellularized ovine rumen reinforced with synthetic interwoven propylene (reinforced biosynthetic ovine rumen, RBOR). This reinforced tissue matrix attempts to combine the benefits of biologic material and polymer reinforcement to provide a more physiologic hernia repair when compared with mesh products composed of just synthetic polymer materials [29]. The synthetic component of this mesh is thought to confer increased long-term strength and load-sharing capacity, while the biologic ovine rumen aims to promote tissue integration, minimize foreign body response, and reduce potential infection by shielding the synthetic component. Biologic matrices derived from porcine or bovine dermis are also employed in contaminated settings, but their high cost and variable long-term outcomes have limited their widespread adoption. Biosynthetic meshes, on the other hand, offer a compromise between mechanical performance and bioresorbability, with lower cost and more predictable manufacturing characteristics. An additional advantage of biosynthetic materials lies in their higher tolerance to postoperative complications. Their complete resorbability can obviate the need for mesh explantation in the event of infection, as the material is gradually degraded and replaced by native connective tissue. However, for optimal integration and a controlled inflammatory response, it is crucial that implantation occurs in a well-vascularized, tension-free plane [30]. Recent clinical guidelines, including the Ventral Hernia Working Group (VHWG) grading scale, recommend biosynthetic meshes for patients classified as Grade III and IV (active contamination, infection, fistula), while permanent synthetic meshes remain appropriate for Grade I and II patients. Nevertheless, high-level evidence remains limited, with much of the current data derived from retrospective series or selected cohorts. Ongoing randomized controlled trials aim to provide definitive long-term comparative outcomes between biosynthetic and permanent synthetic meshes in high-risk surgical contexts [31, 32].

References

1. Muysoms FE, Miserez M, Berrevoet F, et al. Classification of primary and incisional abdominal wall hernias. Hernia. 2009;13(4):407–14.
2. Parker SG, Halligan S, Blackburn S, et al. What exactly is meant by "loss of domain" for ventral hernia? Systematic review of definitions. World J Surg. 2019;43(2):396–404.
3. Campanelli G. The art of hernia surgery. 1st ed. Cham: Springer; 2018.
4. Latifi R. Surgery of complex abdominal wall defects. 2nd ed. Cham: Springer; 2017.
5. Bueno-Lledó J, Torregrosa A, Ballester N, et al. Preoperative progressive pneumoperitoneum and botulinum toxin type A in patients with large incisional hernia. Hernia. 2017;21(2):233–43.
6. Martínez-Hoed J, Bonafe-Diana S, Bueno-Lledó J. A systematic review of the use of progressive preoperative pneumoperitoneum since its inception. Hernia. 2021;25(6):1443–58.
7. Ramaswamy A. Preoperative optimization for abdominal wall reconstruction. Surg Clin North Am. 2023;103(5):917–33.
8. Giuffrida M, Biolchini F, Capelli P, et al. Botulinum toxin and progressive pneumoperitoneum in loss of domain ventral hernias: a systematic review. J Abdom Wall Surg. 2024;3:12650.
9. Tashkandi A, Bueno-Lledó J, Durtette-Guzylack J, et al. Adjunct botox to preoperative progressive pneumoperitoneum for incisional hernia with loss of domain: no additional effect but may improve outcomes. Hernia. 2021;25(6):1507–17.
10. Tanaka EY, Yoo JH, Rodrigues AJ Jr, et al. A computerized tomography scan method for calculating the hernia sac and abdominal cavity volume in complex large incisional hernia with loss of domain. Hernia. 2010;14(1):63–9.
11. Sabbagh C, Dumont F, Robert B, et al. Peritoneal volume is predictive of tension-free fascia closure of large incisional hernias with loss of domain: a prospective study. Hernia. 2011;15(5):559–65.
12. Love MW, Warren JA, Davis S, et al. Computed tomography imaging in ventral hernia repair: can we predict the need for myofascial release? Hernia. 2021;25(2):471–7.
13. Tastaldi L, Krpata DM, Prabhu AS, et al. The effect of increasing body mass index on wound complications in open ventral hernia repair with mesh. Am J Surg. 2019;218(3):560–6.

14. Turmine J, Florence AM, Tardivon C, et al. Obesity increases the surgical complexity and risk of recurrence after midline primary ventral hernia repair: results on 2307 patients from the French Society of hernia surgery (SFCP-CH) registry database. Hernia. 2024;28(3):779–88.
15. Chandeze MM, Moszkowicz D, Beauchet A, et al. Ventral hernia surgery in morbidly obese patients, immediate or after bariatric surgery preparation: results of a case-matched study. Surg Obes Relat Dis. 2019;15(1):83–8.
16. Louis-Gaubert C, de Montrichard M, Jacobi D, et al. Morbidity and mortality of incisional hernia repairs in patients with obesity: a retrospective bicentric study on the impact of an initial bariatric surgery approach. Surg Obes Relat Dis. 2025;21(9):1004–10.
17. Deerenberg EB, Henriksen NA, Antoniou GA, et al. Updated guideline for closure of abdominal wall incisions from the European and American Hernia Societies. Br J Surg. 2022;109(12):1239–50.
18. Li J, Wang Y, Wu L. The comparison of eTEP and IPOM in ventral and incisional hernia repair: a systematic review and meta-analysis. Surg Laparosc Endosc Percutan Tech. 2022;32(2):252–8.
19. Ramirez OM, Ruas E, Dellon AL. "Components separation" method for closure of abdominal-wall defects: an anatomic and clinical study. Plast Reconstr Surg. 1990;86(3):519–26.
20. Kesicioglu T, Yildirim K, Yuruker S, et al. Three-year outcome after anterior component separation repair of giant ventral hernias: a retrospective analysis of the original technique without mesh. Asian J Surg. 2022;45(5):1117–21.
21. Jørgensen LN, Jensen KK. Endoscopic anterior component separation: how we do it? Int J Abdom Wall Hernia Surg. 2022;5(1):8–12.
22. Campanelli G, Bastazza M, Ruca A, et al. Surgical treatment of incisional hernias with marked loss of substance. Hernia. 2000;4:202–5.
23. Novitsky YW, Elliott HL, Orenstein SB, Rosen MJ. Transversus abdominis muscle release: a novel approach to posterior component separation during complex abdominal wall reconstruction. Am J Surg. 2012;204(5):709–16.
24. Cavalli M, Bruni PG, Lombardo F, et al. Original concepts in anatomy, abdominal-wall surgery, and component separation technique and strategy. Hernia. 2020;24(2):411–9.
25. Gandhi JA, Gajjar AP, Shinde PH, Chaudhari S. Posterior component separation technique—original transversus abdominis release (TAR) technique. J Abdom Wall Surg. 2024;3:12542.
26. Cornette B, De Bacquer D, Berrevoet F. Component separation technique for giant incisional hernia: a systematic review. Am J Surg. 2018;215(4):719–26.
27. Bueno-Lledó J, Bonafe-Diana S, Carbonell-Tatay F, et al. Component separation and large incisional hernia: predictive factors of recurrence. Hernia. 2021;25(6):1593–600.
28. Gossetti F, D'amore L, Grimaldi MR, et al. Rives-Stoppa repair of incisional hernias using PVDF mesh: a 10-year experience of a dedicated surgical team. JSM Gastroenterol Hepatol. 2023;10(1):1115.
29. Özant A, Arslan K. Synthetic meshes in hernia surgery. Cyprus J Med Sci. 2023;8:1–7.
30. Sivaraj D, Fischer KS, Kim TS, et al. Outcomes of biosynthetic and synthetic mesh in ventral hernia repair. Plast Reconstr Surg Glob Open. 2022;10(12):e4707.
31. Rognoni C, Bassi UA, Cataldo M, et al. Budget impact analysis of a biosynthetic mesh for incisional hernia repair. Clin Ther. 2018;40(11):1830–44.e4.
32. Charleux-Muller D, Hurel R, Fabacher T, et al. Slowly absorbable mesh in contaminated incisional hernia repair: results of a French multicenter study. Hernia. 2021;25(4):1051–9.

Surgical Techniques for Complex Abdominal Hernias: Open Approach—Techniques, Mesh Placement Options, and Advanced Reconstructive Approaches

7

Laura Roman Garcia de Leon, Joaquin Manuel Muñoz Rodriguez, Javier Lopez Monclus, Luis Blazquez Hernando, Alvaro Robin Valle de Lersundi, Manuel Medina Pedrique, Marcello de Luca, and Miguel Angel Garcia Ureña

7.1 Introduction and Historical Perspective

Hernia repair has experienced remarkable evolution over the past decades, driven by a deeper understanding of anatomy, biomechanics, and the biology of hernia formation and recurrence. Techniques have shifted from simple closure strategies to complex reconstructive procedures that aim not only to repair the defect but also to restore abdominal wall function.

Primary suture repairs were widely used in the early era of abdominal wall surgery but were associated with alarmingly high recurrence rates, reaching up to 50–57% in some series [1]. The introduction of tension-free mesh repair marked a major advancement, although recurrence and complications remained a challenge in complex cases.

In the 1970s, René Stoppa, Jean Rives, and George Wantz pioneered the concept of retromuscular-preperitoneal mesh placement, laying the foundation for what would later be known as the Rives-Stoppa repair or giant prosthetic reinforcement

L. Roman Garcia de Leon (✉) · J. M. Muñoz Rodriguez · J. Lopez Monclus
Department of Abdominal Wall Surgery, Hospital Universitario Puerta de Hierro Majadahonda, Madrid, Spain
e-mail: laura.rgdl@gmail.com

L. Blazquez Hernando
Department of Abdominal Wall Surgery, Hospital Universitario Ramón y Cajal, Madrid, Spain

A. Robin Valle de Lersundi · M. Medina Pedrique · M. de Luca · M. A. Garcia Ureña
Department of Abdominal Wall Surgery, Hospital Universitario del Henares, Madrid, Spain

D. Cuccurullo, C. Rispoli (eds.), *Complex Abdominal Wall Surgery*, Updates in Surgery, https://doi.org/10.1007/978-3-032-24284-6_7

of the visceral sac (GPRVS). This technique involved extensive dissection of the extraperitoneal space and the placement of a large mesh, relying on intra-abdominal pressure for stabilization. It showed excellent outcomes in terms of recurrence and mesh integration [2, 3].

The adaptation of this concept to incisional hernias through the Rives-Stoppa repair became the gold standard for open midline hernia repair, offering robust structural support and low recurrence rates [4].

However, this approach had anatomical limitations, particularly in large or complex hernias where insufficient medial advancement of the rectus muscles was possible due to the constraint of the lateral rectus sheath insertion. To address this, component separation techniques were introduced as an alternative to enhance myofascial mobilization.

The first component separation technique was described by Ramírez et al. in 1990, who introduced the anterior component separation by releasing the external oblique aponeurosis to allow medial mobilization of the myofascial complex [5]. This technique underwent several refinements and expanded the possibilities of closure in large defects.

In 2006, Heniford's group described an open preperitoneal approach for giant hernias, which provided the groundwork for the introduction of the posterior component separation with transversus abdominis release (TAR) by Novitsky et al. in 2012. This technique represented a major step forward: it enabled lateral extension of the retromuscular plane while preserving the neurovascular bundles and avoiding subcutaneous dissection [6, 7].

TAR also expanded the indications for posterior repair by enabling the treatment of defects located near bony boundaries, such as the costal margin or iliac crest, and those involving the lateral abdominal wall. Since its description, numerous modifications of the TAR technique have been published, further improving anatomical precision and clinical outcomes in complex abdominal wall reconstructions.

This progressive technical development has dramatically expanded the armamentarium of abdominal wall surgeons, while also redefining the role of open surgery in the current era—where advanced minimally invasive approaches increasingly coexist with traditional open techniques.

7.2 The Role of Open Surgery in the Current Era

Despite the growing popularity of minimally invasive techniques, open abdominal wall repair continues to play a pivotal role in the management of complex hernias. The last two decades have witnessed the emergence and refinement of laparoscopic and robotic approaches, particularly retromuscular and preperitoneal repairs, which aim to replicate the principles of open surgery while minimizing tissue trauma.

Minimally invasive techniques have gained popularity in recent years, providing alternative approaches that aim to reproduce the advantages of open retromuscular repair while reducing surgical trauma. While the intraperitoneal onlay mesh (IPOM) technique initiated this trend in the early 1990s, it had limitations in complex cases owing to its intraperitoneal nature [8]. The introduction of the extended-view totally extraperitoneal repair eTEP approach in 2012 and the subsequent adoption of robotic platforms significantly expanded the applicability of minimally invasive Rives-Stoppa, preperitoneal, and TAR repairs [9–11]. These advances now coexist with open techniques as complementary tools, each with its own indications and technical requirements. Nevertheless, minimally invasive abdominal wall reconstruction remains technically demanding, often requiring extensive experience, dedicated training, and access to advanced equipment. These approaches are generally concentrated in high-volume referral centers with specialized surgical teams [12].

In contrast, open repair remains a versatile and reproducible approach, particularly in the following contexts:

- Massive or loss of domain hernias;
- Multiple prior repairs or hostile abdomens;
- Hernias associated with infection, fistulas, or skin grafts;
- Lateral and suprapubic hernias near bony or fixed landmarks;
- Emergency settings or when access to minimally invasive tools is limited.

Thus, open abdominal wall reconstruction continues to be essential, particularly in complex or borderline cases where minimally invasive access is unsafe or unfeasible. Instead of being replaced, open techniques are now integrated into a complementary surgical strategy, allowing tailored, patient-centered decision-making.

7.3 Mesh Placement Planes in Open Hernia Repair

The anatomical plane chosen for mesh implantation is a critical factor in determining the success of ventral hernia repair. Different locations offer varying levels of biomechanical support, tissue integration, and complication profiles. Historically, terminology has been inconsistent, hindering communication and comparison across studies. To address this, the International Classification of Abdominal Wall Planes (ICAP) was developed by consensus in 2020, providing a standardized framework to describe mesh positions in relation to the abdominal wall layers [13].

In open surgery, the most frequently utilized planes include (Fig. 7.1):

- *Onlay*: The mesh is placed between the anterior rectus sheath and the subcutaneous tissue. It is technically straightforward and easily accessible but is associated with a higher risk of seroma and surgical site infection.
- *Inlay*: The mesh is sutured directly to the edges of the fascial defect without overlap. It provides minimal biomechanical support and is typically reserved for emergency settings or as a salvage option due to its high recurrence rate.
- *Retrorectus (retromuscular) plane*: Located between the rectus abdominis muscle and the posterior rectus sheath, this is the preferred plane in Rives-Stoppa repairs and is considered the gold standard in open hernia surgery. Its lateral extension requires a TAR to access the space superficial to the transversalis fascia.

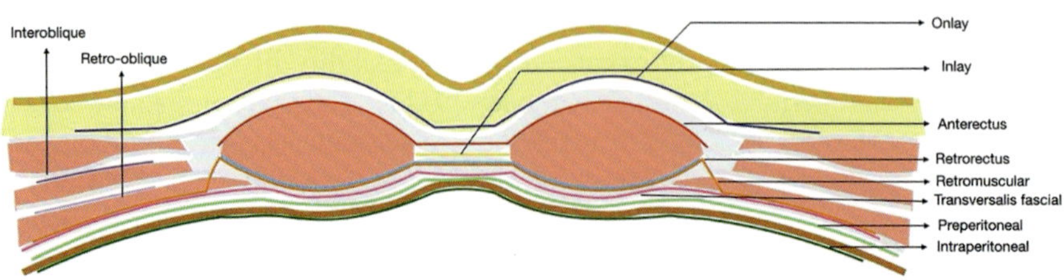

Fig. 7.1 Illustrative summary of the abdominal wall planes, adapted from the Delphi consensus on anatomical classification

- *Transversalis fascial plane*: This space lies immediately cranial to the transversalis fascia. In regions where the posterior rectus sheath is present, it is located just posterior to it; laterally, it is found between the transversus abdominis muscle and the transversalis fascia. This plane has gained relevance with the advent of minimally invasive approaches, although its development via open surgery remains technically challenging.
- *Intraperitoneal plane*: The mesh is placed inside the peritoneal cavity, in direct contact with abdominal viscera. Although occasionally used in emergency or contaminated settings, this location is associated with long-term complications such as adhesions, erosion, and fistula formation, and is generally avoided in elective open repairs.

7.4 Main Open Techniques

7.4.1 Onlay Repair

7.4.1.1 Introduction/Definition

The onlay technique involves the placement of a synthetic mesh over the anterior rectus sheath, between it and the subcutaneous tissue. It is one of the earliest mesh-based techniques used for ventral hernia repair [14].

7.4.1.2 Main Indications

Onlay repair is generally reserved for cases where dissection of deeper planes is contraindicated or unfeasible, such as in contaminated fields, hostile abdomens, or when simpler approaches are preferred due to patient comorbidities.

7.4.1.3 Surgical Technique (Step-by-Step)

After exposure of the hernia defect and reduction of its contents, the subcutaneous tissue is dissected widely to expose the anterior rectus sheath and create space for adequate mesh overlap (typically at least 5 cm). The fascial defect is then closed primarily to restore midline continuity. The mesh is positioned over the anterior sheath and fixed using sutures—either absorbable or non-absorbable—according to surgeon preference. Atraumatic fixation methods, such as fibrin glue or cyanoacrylate adhesives, have also been described and may reduce postoperative pain and seroma formation [15, 16]. One or more suction drains are typically placed to minimize fluid accumulation.

7.4.1.4 Advantages and Limitations

The onlay technique is technically simple and does not require deep dissection, making it accessible in many surgical settings. However, it carries a higher risk of seroma, surgical site infection, and mesh-related complications due to its proximity to the skin. Recurrence rates may also be higher compared to sublay techniques [17].

7.4.2 Chevrel Repair

7.4.2.1 Introduction/Definition

The Chevrel technique is a modification of the onlay repair that incorporates a sliding myofascial advancement flap to achieve tension-free closure of the midline. First described in the 1970s by Jacques Chevrel, it involves longitudinal incisions in the anterior rectus sheath to allow medialization of the rectus muscles before mesh placement [18].

7.4.2.2 Main Indications

This approach is particularly useful in midline hernias with moderate loss of domain where fascial closure under tension is not feasible with a simple onlay or primary suture. It is also indicated in recurrent hernias where sublay planes are not accessible due to prior surgery.

7.4.2.3 Surgical Technique (Step-by-Step)

After dissection of the subcutaneous tissue and exposure of the anterior rectus sheath, longitudinal incisions are made along the medial edge of each sheath to create sliding myofascial flaps. This allows for medial advancement of the rectus muscles and facilitates primary closure of the midline without tension, when feasible. A mesh is then placed in the onlay position over the reinforced fascia and fixed using either absorbable or non-absorbable sutures. Atraumatic fixation with fibrin glue has also been proposed in selected cases to reduce complications. Drains are routinely placed to reduce the risk of seroma formation [19, 20].

7.4.2.4 Advantages and Limitations

The Chevrel repair allows for effective midline closure even in large defects and is technically simpler than component separation techniques. However, it shares many of the drawbacks of the onlay position, including higher risks of seroma and wound complications. Its use has declined in favor of sublay and retromuscular approaches in recent years [21].

7.4.3 Rives-Stoppa

7.4.3.1 Introduction/Definition

The Rives-Stoppa technique represents a cornerstone in modern open abdominal wall reconstruction. Initially described by René Stoppa for the repair of large inguinal hernias, the technique involved extensive dissection of the preperitoneal space and the placement of a large, unfixated mesh, relying on intra-abdominal pressure to maintain positioning—the so-called "Giant Prosthetic Reinforcement of the Visceral Sac" (GPRVS) [3]. Jean Rives extended the concept to the retromuscular plane for midline ventral hernias, facilitating mesh placement between the rectus abdominis muscle and the posterior rectus sheath above the arcuate line. George Wantz subsequently popularized the technique in the United States [2].

Together, these pioneers laid the anatomical and conceptual foundation of what would later be recognized as the first true fascial release, predating the formalization of component separation techniques. The Rives-Stoppa approach evolved into the gold standard for midline hernia repairs of small to moderate size, offering excellent functional and anatomical results with low recurrence and complication rates [22].

7.4.3.2 Main Indications

This technique is particularly suitable for midline hernias with defects up to 10 cm, as demonstrated by Stoppa's early biomechanical studies [3]. The retromuscular plane is highly vascularized, promoting mesh integration while distancing the prosthesis from intra-abdominal viscera and avoiding the complications associated with subcutaneous dissection. Rives-Stoppa repair enables restoration of the linea alba and strong fascial closure with favorable outcomes in terms of durability, infection, and recurrence [4].

7.4.3.3 Surgical Technique (Step-by-Step)

- *Hernia Sac Management*: Following skin incision, the hernia sac is opened to facilitate visualization and control of its contents. The sac is preserved until late in the procedure to assist in posterior and anterior layer reconstruction if needed. This maneuver, wherein the sac is divided and used to reinforce both fascial layers, is referred to as the peritoneal flap repair [23, 24].
- *Adhesiolysis*: The hernia contents are reduced, and adhesiolysis is performed to separate intra-abdominal structures from the anterior abdominal wall, minimizing the risk of visceral injury during dissection [25].
- *Posterior rectus sheath and retromuscular dissection* (Fig. 7.2): The posterior rectus sheath is incised as close as possible to its medial border. Blunt dissection is carried out between the rectus abdominis muscle and the posterior sheath, carefully preserving the neurovascular bundles located laterally. Dissection is extended laterally to the lateral reflection of the posterior sheath and continued in a craniocaudal direction along both rectus compartments. In the midline, the preperitoneal plane is maintained, following the medial prong of the fatty trident

[26]. The medial edge of both posterior rectus sheaths is incised to unify the space dissected.

- *Preperitoneal dissection below the arcuate line*: Caudal to the arcuate line, where the posterior rectus sheath is absent, dissection continues in the true preperitoneal plane over the preperitoneal fat or transversalis fascia [27]. The caudal limit is the pubic tubercle and Cooper's ligaments. In defects near the pubis, dissection may be extended beyond these landmarks.
- *Cranial extension and the fatty trident* (Fig. 7.3): Cranially, following the original description by Stoppa and later highlighted by García Ureña et al., the medial incision of the posterior rectus sheath should be discontinued approximately 6 cm below the xiphoid process, as continuing the dissection beyond this point would lead above the costal margins. At this level, the posterior sheath must be transversely incised to allow for a change in dissection plane [28]. Dissection then proceeds between the posterior rectus sheath and the transversalis fascia laterally, while the preperitoneal plane is preserved in the midline. This central space expands into a fat-filled rhomboid area, and a fat pad—previously referred to as the "fatty triangle"—must be left attached to the xiphoid. Dissection should generally stop at the xiphoid level unless the hernia defect extends more cranially, in which case the dissection may be continued into the subdiaphragmatic space to ensure adequate overlap.
- *Closure of posterior layer*: The posterior sheath and/or peritoneum are closed with long-lasting absorbable sutures. If tension is present, a peritoneal or omental patch may be used. If this is not feasible, bridging of the layer with absorbable material or lateral extension via component separation may be performed [29, 30].
- *Mesh placement*: A large, permanent mesh is placed in the retromuscular plane to cover the entire dissected area.
- *Mesh fixation*: Originally performed with non-absorbable sutures, current evidence supports the use of long-lasting absorbable or even atraumatic fixation with glue. In cases of adequate overlap and proper preperitoneal positioning,

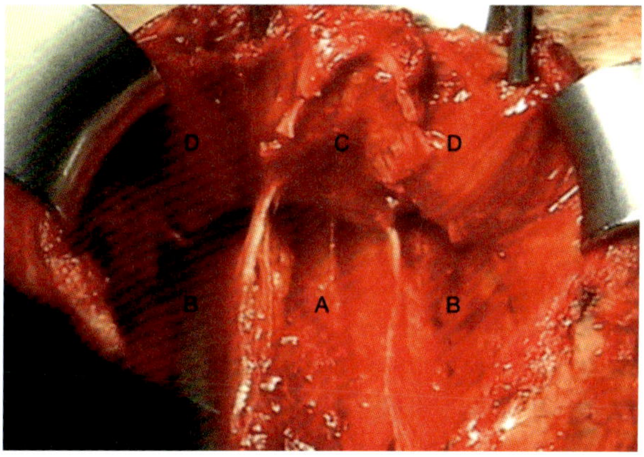

Fig. 7.2 Dissection image of a Rives-Stoppa repair. (**a**) Preperitoneal fat at the midline; (**b**) Posterior rectus sheath; (**c**) Linea alba; (**d**) Rectus muscle

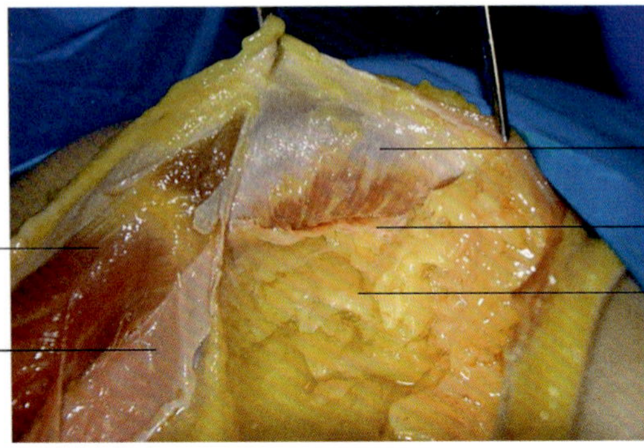

Fig. 7.3 Transition of dissection plane approximately 6 cm below the xiphoid, leaving the posterior rectus sheath (PRS) and transversus abdominis muscle (TAM) attached above, and continuing in the preperitoneal/pretransversalis plane

fixation may be omitted following Stoppa's principle of pressure stabilization [31].

- *Closure of the anterior sheath*: The anterior rectus sheath is closed with long-term absorbable sutures. In cases of tension or tissue loss, bridging or further myofascial advancement may be necessary.
- *Drains*: Suction drains are not routinely used, but they may be placed in the retromuscular or subcutaneous space, particularly if extensive dissection was performed.

7.4.3.4 Advantages and Limitations

The Rives-Stoppa technique remains one of the most effective and physiologically sound repairs for ventral hernias. It allows for tension-free closure with an extraperitoneal prosthesis in a well-vascularized compartment, excellent biomechanical reinforcement, and minimal contact with viscera. The technique is reproducible and versatile but requires extensive anatomical knowledge, can be technically demanding in the upper abdominal region due to mediastinal proximity, and may be limited in defects with insufficient lateral space or prior retromuscular violation.

7.4.4 Anterior Component Separation

7.4.4.1 Introduction/Definition

The anterior component separation (ACS) technique was introduced by Ramírez et al. in 1990 as a means to achieve medial advancement of the abdominal wall by releasing the external oblique aponeurosis [5]. This allows for significant mobilization of the myofascial complex, facilitating tension-free closure of large midline defects. ACS marked a turning point in hernia surgery, laying the groundwork for modern concepts of dynamic abdominal wall reconstruction.

7.4.4.2 Main Indications

ACS is particularly useful in large midline hernias where primary fascial closure is not possible despite extensive retromuscular dissection. It is indicated when defects exceed the closure capacity of posterior repairs or when additional medialization is needed to restore functional continuity of the abdominal wall. ACS may also be considered in recurrent hernias or in cases with prior violation of the retromuscular plane [32].

7.4.4.3 Surgical Technique (Step-by-Step)

- *Dissection of subcutaneous tissue*: After midline exposure and reduction of the hernia, bilateral subcutaneous flaps are elevated to expose the external oblique aponeurosis.
- *External oblique release*: The aponeurosis is incised longitudinally approximately 2 cm lateral to the medial convergence of the oblique musculature (traditionally referred to as the linea semilunaris, but more recently described as the EIT *ambivium*) [33]. Care is taken to preserve the internal oblique muscle and its neurovascular bundles [34].
- *Myofascial advancement*: The external oblique muscle is dissected free from the underlying internal oblique, enabling medial advancement of the rectus-internal oblique-transversus complex by up to 10 cm in the upper abdomen and 5–7 cm in the lower abdomen.
- *Fascial closure and mesh reinforcement*: Following adequate medialization, the midline fascia is closed and reinforced with a mesh, typically placed in a retrorectus or onlay position, depending on the feasibility of posterior layer reconstruction.
- *Modifications*:
  - *Perforator-sparing technique:* This technique preserves periumbilical perforating vessels to reduce the risk of flap necrosis [35].
  - *Endoscopic anterior component separation:* This minimally invasive approach enables division of the external oblique aponeurosis through small incisions, reducing wound complications while preserving advancement [36].

7.4.4.4 Advantages and Limitations

ACS allows for substantial medial advancement and facilitates closure of large defects, making it a valuable option in complex reconstructions. However, it requires wide subcutaneous dissection, which increases the risk of wound complications, seroma, and skin ischemia. Perforator-sparing and endoscopic modifications may mitigate these risks but demand greater technical precision [5, 37, 38].

7.4.5 Open Preperitoneal Repair

7.4.5.1 Introduction/Definition

Open preperitoneal repair was first described by the Heniford group in 2006 as an alternative technique for ventral hernia repair using a posterior approach [7]. This technique involves wide dissection of the preperitoneal space, allowing for extraperitoneal mesh placement without entering the retromuscular plane. Although initially underutilized, it has recently gained renewed interest as the development of minimally invasive surgery has improved understanding of the preperitoneal space, thereby contributing to its resurgence in open hernia repair [10, 39, 40].

7.4.5.2 Main Indications

This technique is indicated for the treatment of ventral hernias. Its "ideal" indication remains to be clearly defined, though theoretically, it should be applicable to any patient considered for a posterior approach. Because its adoption was limited until recently, specific indications are not yet well established. It may be particularly useful in cases of recurrent hernias, lateral defects, or in patients with compromised retromuscular planes due to prior surgeries [41].

7.4.5.3 Surgical Technique (Step-by-Step)

- *Access and hernia sac management*: The skin is incised along previous scars, and the hernia sac is managed similarly to retromuscular techniques. The sac should be preserved when possible in case it is needed to bridge a posterior or anterior fascial defect.
- *Preperitoneal plane creation*: The dissection is performed predominantly bluntly, using the surgeon's finger, in a circumferential manner [7]. It begins by opening the space of Retzius and exposing both Cooper's ligaments. The dissection is then extended laterally, following the distribution of preperitoneal fat in a trident configuration [26], and cranially toward the subdiaphragmatic region and xiphoid process. Finally, the dissection continues medially, which is often the most technically challenging area. Any peritoneal defects should be closed with sutures or patched using omentum or preserved hernia sac [7, 41].
- *Mesh placement*: A synthetic mesh is placed throughout the dissected preperitoneal space. The mesh lies beneath the muscular plane and the posterior rectus sheath in the medial area. It is typically held in place by intra-abdominal pressure and does not usually require fixation if adequate overlap is achieved.
- *Closure*: The anterior fascia is closed over the mesh using long-lasting absorbable sutures. Suction drains are not routinely used but may be placed if deemed necessary, particularly in cases involving extensive dissection.

7.4.5.4 Advantages and Limitations

Open preperitoneal repair offers a favorable anatomical plane for mesh integration, distant from both viscera and subcutaneous tissues, and avoids the morbidity associated with wide subcutaneous dissection. It also preserves the retromuscular plane for potential future surgeries [41, 42]. However, the dissection can be technically demanding, particularly in thin patients or those with significant adhesions, and requires detailed anatomical knowledge of the preperitoneal space.

7.4.6 Posterior Component Separation (Transversus Abdominis Release)

7.4.6.1 Introduction/Definition

Posterior component separation with transversus abdominis release (TAR) was first described by Novitsky et al. in 2012 and has since become one of the cornerstone techniques in abdominal wall reconstruction. It revolutionized the management of complex ventral hernias by extending the retromuscular dissection laterally, enabling significant medial advancement of the abdominal wall and facilitating the placement of a large prosthetic mesh in the extraperitoneal space [3, 6]. Over time, TAR has gained a central role in abdominal wall reconstruction, offering effective solutions for complex hernias previously considered high risk or challenging to treat [43].

7.4.6.2 Main Indications

TAR is indicated for large or complex midline ventral hernias, including cases with loss of domain, recurrence after prior repairs, and hernias with significant muscular retraction. It is especially useful when the rectus muscles are significantly displaced laterally or when the retrorectal space alone is insufficient to achieve closure [4, 43, 44]. TAR also provides excellent access for lateral hernias and can be combined with other techniques for more extensive reconstructions.

7.4.6.3 Surgical Technique (Step-by-Step)

The initial steps of retromuscular dissection, including opening the posterior rectus sheath and developing the retrorectus plane, have been described in Sect. 7.3 (Rives-Stoppa technique) and are not repeated in detail here.

- *TAR*: Once the retrorectus space is fully developed and the lateral border of the Rives-Stoppa dissection is reached, the need for additional medial advancement is assessed. If required, the posterior rectus sheath is incised laterally, just medial to the neurovascular bundles, to expose the fibers of the transversus abdominis muscle. In the original description by Novitsky, this release is initiated in the upper abdomen, where the transversus abdominis inserts more medially, facilitating plane identification [6, 45]. The muscle fibers are retracted to access the space between the transversus and the transversalis fascia, which is then dissected laterally until reaching the lateral preperitoneal fat. At this point, the dissection transitions to a purely preperitoneal plane. The dissection proceeds craniocaudally, continuing the release of the posterior rectus sheath lateral to the rectus muscle but medial to the neurovascular bundles, extending beyond the arcuate line. In the lower abdomen, once the Bogros space is reached, the dissection reverts to the preperitoneal plane, extending caudally and laterally to visualize the psoas major and quadratus lumborum muscles.

- *Posterior rectus sheath release (Madrid modification)* (Figs. 7.4 and 7.5): Over time, several modifications have been introduced to refine the original TAR technique. The medialization of the transversus abdominis muscle in the upper abdomen brings with it the cranial neurovascular bundles. Dividing the muscle at this level, as originally described, may risk denervation. To avoid this, the Madrid group (García-Ureña et al.) proposed initiating the dissection caudally and advancing cranially, following the myoaponeurotic border of the transversus abdominis [46]. In the cranial portion, the muscle is not divided; instead, the dissection continues by following this anatomical boundary, preserving both the muscle and its neurovascular structures [28, 47].
- *Superior dissection*: Superiorly, dissection can be extended as described in the Rives-Stoppa technique, up to the central tendon of the diaphragm. After identifying the plane between the transversus abdominis muscle and the transversalis fascia, dissection is carried cranially. Transversus fibers interdigitate with the diaphragm near the costal margin, separated by a layer of fat—the so-called "sentinel fat"—which marks the transition between muscle groups [26, 48]. Following this plane allows extension under the diaphragm, providing mesh overlap in subcostal hernias.
- *Inferior dissection*: Inferiorly, dissection follows the same principles as in the Rives-Stoppa technique, extending below Cooper's ligament and continuing preperitoneally into the myopectineal orifice to ensure optimal coverage.
- *Posterior layer reconstruction*: The posterior layer—composed of peritoneum, transversalis fascia, and/or posterior sheath remnants—is closed with long-lasting absorbable sutures. In cases of tension, bridging with preserved hernia sac or omentum may be used. Alternatively, lateral dissection may be extended to facilitate closure.
- *Mesh placement*: A large, synthetic mesh is placed in the retromuscular and pre-transversalis plane, covering the entire dissected area with wide lateral, superior, and inferior overlap. Mesh fixation is usually unnecessary due to the extensive overlap and intraabdominal pressure; however, if fixation is used, it is typically done with two interrupted sutures to Cooper's ligaments [28, 49].

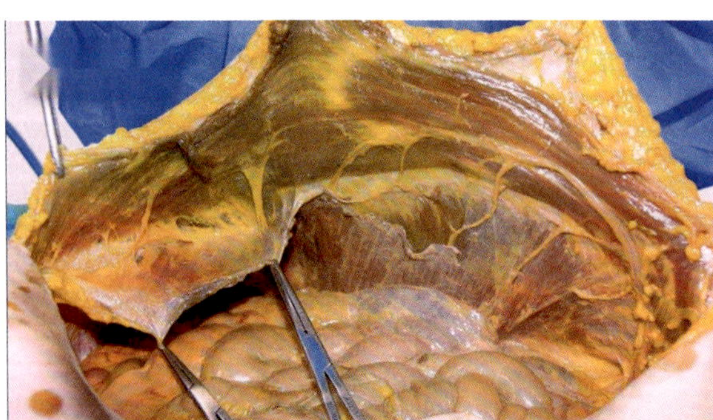

Fig. 7.4 Visualization of the neurovascular bundles following the insertion of the transversus abdominis muscle belly, with medial course in the cranial region

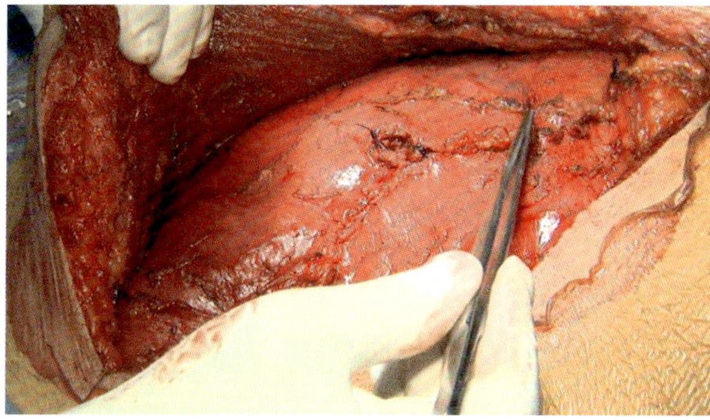

Fig. 7.5 Completely dissected posterior plane, showing medialization of the lateral section of the posterior rectus sheath in the cranial part, following the myoaponeurotic limit of the transversus abdominis muscle

- *Anterior fascia closure and drains*: The final step is the closure of the anterior fascia, aiming to restore the linea alba, particularly relevant in young or physically active patients. When feasible, this is achieved with a primary suture using slowly absorbable monofilament material. However, in cases where tension is excessive or closure is not possible, several alternative strategies have been described. These include bridging techniques, myofascial advancement flaps, and fascial traction devices (e.g., Fasciotens®), which have shown promising but still preliminary results [50, 51]. Additionally, in selected cases where no other option is viable, an associated anterior component separation may be considered to facilitate tension-free closure, despite being more invasive [32]. Suction drains are not routinely used but may be placed in the retromuscular or subcutaneous space, particularly if extensive dissection was performed.

7.4.6.4 Advantages and Limitations

TAR offers extensive myofascial medialization while preserving the integrity of anterior abdominal wall structures. It allows for wide mesh placement in a well-vascularized, extraperitoneal space with minimal risk of bowel contact. This technique facilitates reconstruction of large, complex defects and is versatile across a broad range of hernia scenarios. It also enables posterior closure even in anatomically challenging cases. However, TAR is technically demanding and requires advanced anatomical understanding and surgical expertise. Complications may include seroma, bleeding, or inadvertent injury to neurovascular bundles if not properly identified and preserved.

References

1. Luijendijk RW, Hop WCJ, van den Tol MP, et al. A comparison of suture repair with mesh repair for incisional hernia. N Engl J Med. 2000;343(6):392–8.
2. Wantz GE. Giant prosthetic reinforcement of the visceral sac. Surg Gynecol Obstet. 1989;169(5):408–17.
3. Stoppa RE. The treatment of complicated groin and incisional hernias. World J Surg. 1989;13(5):545–54.

4. Sanders DL, Pawlak MM, Simons MP, et al. Midline incisional hernia guidelines: the European Hernia Society. Br J Surg. 2023;110(12):1732–68.
5. Ramirez OM, Ruas E, Dellon AL. "Components separation" method for closure of abdominal-wall defects. Plast Reconstr Surg. 1990;86(3):519–26.
6. Novitsky YW, Elliott HL, Orenstein SB, Rosen MJ. Transversus abdominis muscle release: a novel approach to posterior component separation during complex abdominal wall reconstruction. Am J Surg. 2012;204(5):709–16.
7. Novitsky YW, Porter JR, Rucho ZC, et al. Open preperitoneal retrofascial mesh repair for multiply recurrent ventral incisional hernias. J Am Coll Surg. 2006;203(3):283–9.
8. LeBlanc KA, Booth WV. Laparoscopic repair of incisional abdominal hernias using expanded polytetrafluoroethylene: preliminary findings. Surg Laparosc Endosc. 1993;3(1):39–41.
9. Belyansky I, Daes J, Radu VG, et al. A novel approach using the enhanced-view totally extraperitoneal (eTEP) technique for laparoscopic retromuscular hernia repair. Surg Endosc. 2018;32(3):1525–32.
10. Belyansky I, Reza Zahiri H, Sanford Z, et al. Early operative outcomes of endoscopic (eTEP access) robotic-assisted retromuscular abdominal wall hernia repair. Hernia. 2018;22(5):837–47.
11. Martin-Del-Campo LA, Weltz AS, Belyansky I, Novitsky YW. Comparative analysis of perioperative outcomes of robotic versus open transversus abdominis release. Surg Endosc. 2018;32(2):840–5.
12. Korneffel K, Nuzzo W, Belden CM, et al. Learning curves of robotic extended totally extraperitoneal (eTEP) hernia repair among two surgeons at a high-volume community hospital: a cumulative sum analysis. Surg Endosc. 2023;37(12):9351–7.
13. Parker SG, Halligan S, Liang MK, et al. International classification of abdominal wall planes (ICAP) to describe mesh insertion for ventral hernia repair. Br J Surg. 2020;107(3):209–17.
14. Köckerling F. Onlay technique in incisional hernia repair—a systematic review. Front Surg. 2018;5:71.
15. Stoikes N, Webb D, Powell B, Voeller G. Preliminary report of a sutureless onlay technique for incisional hernia repair using fibrin glue alone for mesh fixation. Am Surg. 2013;79(11):1177–80.
16. Shahan CP, Stoikes NF, Webb DL, Voeller GR. Sutureless onlay hernia repair: a review of 97 patients. Surg Endosc. 2016;30(8):3256–61.
17. den Hartog D, Dur AHM, Tuinebreijer WE, Kreis RW. Open surgical procedures for incisional hernias. Cochrane Database Syst Rev. 2008;2008(3):CD006438.
18. Chevrel JP. The treatment of large midline incisional hernias by "overcoat" plasty and prothesis (author's transl). Nouv Press Med. 1979;8(9):695–6.
19. Köhler G, Koch OO, Antoniou SA, et al. Prevention of subcutaneous seroma formation in open ventral hernia repair using a new low-thrombin fibrin sealant. World J Surg. 2014;38(11):2797–803.
20. Gurusamy KS, Allen VB. Wound drains after incisional hernia repair. Cochrane Database Syst Rev. 2013;2013(12):CD005570.
21. Köckerling F. What do we know about the Chevrel technique in ventral incisional hernia repair? Front Surg. 2019;6:15.
22. Hartog FPJD, Sneiders D, Darwish EF, et al. Favorable outcomes after retro-rectus (Rives-Stoppa) mesh repair as treatment for noncomplex ventral abdominal wall hernia, a systematic review and meta-analysis. Ann Surg. 2022;276(1):55–65.
23. Malik A, Macdonald ADH, de Beaux AC, Tulloh BR. The peritoneal flap hernioplasty for repair of large ventral and incisional hernias. Hernia. 2014;18(1):39–45.
24. Nielsen MF, de Beaux A, Tulloh B. Peritoneal flap hernioplasty for reconstruction of large ventral hernias: long-term outcome in 251 patients. World J Surg. 2019;43(9):2157–63.
25. Jones CM, Winder JS, Potochny JD, Pauli EM. Posterior component separation with transversus abdominis release. Plast Reconstr Surg. 2016;137(2):636–46.

26. Garcia-Urena MÁ, Lopez-Monclus J, de Robin Valle de Lersundi A, et al. Pathways of the preperitoneal plane: from the "fatty triangle" in Rives to the "fatty trident" in extended retromuscular abdominal wall reconstruction. A tribute to Prof. Schumpelick. Hernia. 2023;27(2):395–407.
27. Henriksen NA, Bougard H, Gonçalves MR, et al. Primary ventral and incisional hernias: comprehensive review. BJS Open. 2024;9(1):zrae145.
28. De Luca M, López-Monclús J, Muñoz-Rodríguez JM, et al. How I do it: Madrid posterior component separation in 10 steps, with special consideration of its anatomy. Langenbecks Arch Surg. 2024;409(1):349.
29. Winder JS, Majumder A, Fayezizadeh M, et al. Outcomes of utilizing absorbable mesh as an adjunct to posterior sheath closure during complex posterior component separation. Hernia. 2018;22(2):303–9.
30. Messer N, Miller BT, Beffa LRA, et al. Outcomes of posterior sheath supplementation with Vicryl mesh in TAR—a single-center study. Hernia. 2024;28(3):905–11.
31. Ellis RC, Petro CC, Krpata DM, et al. Transfascial fixation vs no fixation for open retromuscular ventral hernia repairs: a randomized clinical trial. JAMA Surg. 2023;158(8):789–95.
32. Lopez-Monclus J, Muñoz-Rodríguez J, San Miguel C, et al. Combining anterior and posterior component separation for extreme cases of abdominal wall reconstruction. Hernia. 2020;24(2):369–79.
33. Vierstraete M, Pereira Rodriguez JA, Renard Y, Muysoms F. EIT ambivium, linea semilunaris, and fulcrum abdominalis. J Abdom Wall Surg. 2023;2:12217.
34. Tastaldi L, Alkhatib H. Incisional hernia repair: open retromuscular approaches. Surg Clin North Am. 2018;98(3):511–35.
35. Dumanian GA. Abdominal wall reconstruction. In: Thorne CH, Chung KC, Gosain AK, Gurtner GC, Mehrara BJ, Rubin JP, Spear SL, editors. Grabb and Smith's plastic surgery. 7th ed. Philadelphia: Lippincott Williams & Wilkins; 2013. p. 933–40.
36. Dauser B, Ghaffari S, Ng C, et al. Endoscopic anterior component separation: a novel technical approach. Hernia. 2017;21(6):951–5.
37. Ghali S, Turza KC, Baumann DP, Butler CE. Minimally invasive component separation results in fewer wound-healing complications than open component separation for large ventral hernia repairs. J Am Coll Surg. 2012;214(6):981–9.
38. Gonzalez R, Rehnke RD, Ramaswamy A, et al. Components separation technique and laparoscopic approach: a review of two evolving strategies for ventral hernia repair. Am Surg. 2005;71(7):598–605.
39. Alpuche HAV, Torres FR, González JPS. Early results of eTEP access surgery with preperitoneal repair of primary midline ventral hernias and diastasis recti. A 33 patient case series of "PeTEP". Surg Endosc. 2024;38(6):3204–11.
40. Shao JM, Deerenberg EB, Elhage SA, et al. Are laparoscopic and open ventral hernia repairs truly comparable?: a propensity-matched study in large ventral hernias. Surg Endosc. 2021;35(8):4653–60.
41. Heniford BT, Ross SW, Wormer BA, et al. Preperitoneal ventral hernia repair: a decade long prospective observational study with analysis of 1023 patient outcomes. Ann Surg. 2020;271(2):364–74.
42. Katzen MM, Kercher KW, Sacco JM, et al. Open preperitoneal ventral hernia repair: prospective observational study of quality improvement outcomes over 18 years and 1,842 patients. Surgery. 2023;173(3):739–47.
43. Wegdam JA, Thoolen JMM, Nienhuijs SW, et al. Systematic review of transversus abdominis release in complex abdominal wall reconstruction. Hernia. 2019;23(1):5–15.
44. Zolin SJ, Fafaj A, Krpata DM. Transversus abdominis release (TAR): what are the real indications and where is the limit? Hernia. 2020;24(2):333–40.
45. Gandhi JA, Gajjar AP, Shinde PH, Chaudhari S. Posterior component separation technique—original transversus abdominis release (TAR) technique. J Abdom Wall Surg. 2024;3:12542.

46. Robin-Lersundi A, Blazquez Hernando L, López-Monclús J, et al. How we do it: down to up posterior components separation. Langenbecks Arch Surg. 2018;403(4):539–46.
47. De Luca M, Medina Pedrique M, Morejon Ruiz S, et al. The Madrid posterior component separation: an anatomical approach for effective reconstruction of complex midline hernias. J Abdom Wall Surg. 2024;3:12928.
48. Garcia Ureña MÁ, López-Monclús J, Hernando LAB, et al. Incisional hernia: open abdominal wall reconstruction. Current state of the technique and results. Chirurgie (Heidelb). 2024;95(1):10–9.
49. Weltz AS, Sibia US, Zahiri HR, et al. Operative outcomes after open abdominal wall reconstruction with retromuscular mesh fixation using fibrin glue versus transfascial sutures. Am Surg. 2017;83(9):937–42.
50. Niebuhr H, Wegner F, Dag H, et al. Preoperative botolinum toxin A (BTA) and intraoperative fascial traction (IFT) in the management of complex abdominal wall hernias. Hernia. 2024;28(6):2273–83.
51. Niebuhr H, Aufenberg T, Dag H, et al. Intraoperative fascia tension as an alternative to component separation. A prospective observational study. Front Surg. 2021;7:616669.

Laparo-Endoscopic Approaches for Complex Abdominal Hernias

8

Salvador Morales-Conde, Veronica Tamburi, and Andrea Balla

8.1 Introduction

The management of complex abdominal wall hernias represents one of the most demanding challenges in modern hernia surgery. Despite significant advances in the knowledge of the anatomy and surgical prosthetic materials and techniques, these hernias remain associated with high recurrence rates, morbidity, and a major impact on patients' quality of life. The term "complex hernia" encompasses a broad spectrum of abdominal wall defects that cannot be treated with standard techniques owing to their size, location, soft tissue conditions, such as infection, fistulas or excess of skin, or patient-related factors.

The definition of a "complex" abdominal wall hernia has evolved significantly over the past decade. Recently, the European Hernia Society (EHS) refined and expanded this definition through a Delphi consensus study published in the British Journal of Surgery in 2024 [1]. This updated consensus emphasizes a multidimensional approach, integrating not only anatomical and technical factors but also systemic, patient-specific, and contextual elements, such as comorbidities, functional impairment, and previous abdominal wall reconstruction. The EHS consensus thus establishes a comprehensive framework for defining complexity, acknowledging that it extends beyond mere defect size to encompass biological and functional challenges.

Before starting to analyze the surgical strategy, it is important to state, that not all complex hernias should be surgically treated. Decision-making must balance operative risk, patient comorbidities, and the expected functional and aesthetic benefits. In selected cases, conservative management or delayed reconstruction may yield better long-term outcomes than immediate repair.

S. Morales-Conde (✉) · V. Tamburi · A. Balla
Department of General and Digestive Surgery, University Hospital Virgen Macarena, University of Sevilla, Sevilla, Spain
e-mail: smoralesc@gmail.com; veronicatamburi.94@gmail.com; andrea.balla@gmail.com

D. Cuccurullo, C. Rispoli (eds.), *Complex Abdominal Wall Surgery*, Updates in Surgery, https://doi.org/10.1007/978-3-032-24284-6_8

In this chapter, we focus on laparo-endoscopic techniques for the repair of complex ventral and incisional hernias. These minimally invasive approaches have evolved, driven by the goal of reducing surgical trauma while maintaining durable and functional repairs. Laparo-endoscopic repair also offers in complex hernias several advantages: reduced wound complications, shorter hospital stay, lower postoperative pain, and faster recovery compared with open reconstruction [2]. Additionally, the enhanced visualization of the abdominal wall allows for precise identification of the anatomy, dissection and mesh placement, particularly valuable in recurrences and cases in the lateral abdomen or close to the bone margins. Recent innovations in hybrid and robotic-assisted techniques have further expanded the role of minimally invasive surgery in complex abdominal wall repair [3].

However, minimally invasive repair is not universally suitable. Very large defects with significant loss of domain, infected meshes, or concomitant enterocutaneous fistulas remain best managed with open or staged approaches. Patient selection is essential, as well as anatomical feasibility and surgeon expertise, in order to achieve safe and durable outcomes.

The objective of this chapter is to provide a comprehensive yet practical overview of laparo-endoscopic strategies in the management of complex ventral and incisional hernias, emphasizing their specific role within modern abdominal wall reconstruction. In accordance with the structure of this volume, we will not cover topics extensively discussed in other chapters, such as preoperative optimization. Likewise, large hernias and cases with soft-tissue involvement (infection, fistulas, skin redundancy), or patients with comorbid conditions that significantly alter outcomes (such as severe obesity) will be excluded from the present discussion. Instead, this chapter will concentrate on the principles, operative details, and outcomes of laparo-endoscopic procedures, aiming to offer an evidence-based guide for the contemporary hernia surgeon, as well as the management of those hernias located in complex locations.

As abdominal wall surgery continues to evolve, the integration of minimally invasive and robotic approaches represents a paradigm shift toward precision, functionality, and patient-centered outcomes. Through careful application and continuous research, these techniques have the potential to redefine standards in complex hernia management.

8.2 Evolution of Laparo-Endoscopic Techniques for Ventral Hernia Repair

The evolution of laparo-endoscopic techniques for ventral hernia repair represents a significant shift in abdominal wall surgery over the past three decades. The journey began with the introduction of the intraperitoneal onlay mesh (IPOM) technique by LeBlanc in the early 1990s [4], which provided a minimally invasive alternative to conventional open repair by placing a prosthetic mesh intraperitoneally through a laparoscopic approach. Although IPOM and its alternatives with new fixation methods, such as the "double crown" [5] promoted by our group, rapidly gained popularity due to their reduced wound morbidity, faster recovery, and shorter hospital stay, their limitations soon became evident [2]. The defect was not closed, the mesh was in direct contact with intra-abdominal viscera, and the necessary fixation led to problems such as pain and bulging. Despite these drawbacks, IPOM established the conceptual foundation for minimally invasive ventral hernia surgery. The next milestone was the concept of IPOM-Plus [6], which incorporated defect closure before placing the intra-abdominal mesh, improving functional outcomes and reducing complications, decreasing the risk of seroma and bulging.

More recently, with growing fear of having a prosthetic material in contact with the bowel and an increasing understanding of abdominal wall anatomy, retromuscular approaches were developed. Extended totally extraperitoneal (eTEP) [7] repairs, the transabdominal retromuscular approach (Lap sublay) [8] and access through the hernia defect (e-MILOS) [9] aimed to recreate the sublay plane of open Rives-Stoppa repairs but through a minimally invasive approach, thereby combining the advantages of laparoscopy (smaller incisions, less pain, fewer wound complications) with the durability of an anatomical mesh position. These approaches represented a paradigm shift, allowing wide retromuscular dissection and large mesh placement.

The laparo-endoscopic component separation [10] further expanded the scope of minimally invasive surgery by allowing myofascial release through small incisions, significantly reducing wound complications in large hernias more than 10 cm. Over the past decade, these approaches have been refined with improved visualization, energy devices, and ergonomic instrumentation.

Recently, as an alternative to the large and technically demanding dissection required for retromuscular repairs, preperitoneal approaches have emerged that offer, in selected cases, a more physiological option that does not invade the retromuscular plane. The so-called ventral transabdominal preperitoneal (TAPP) repair [11] involves entering the peritoneal cavity and developing a preperitoneal space by a laparoscopic approach. Once the defect is closed, a large polypropylene mesh is placed in this space with generous overlap, followed by peritoneal closure with a continuous suture to fully isolate the prosthesis from the viscera.

This technique reproduces the concept of an extraperitoneal reconstruction without the need for extensive posterior sheath release, reducing the technical difficulty and minimizing postoperative hematomas. Building on this idea, a purely extraperitoneal variant—the peritoneal-endoscopic totally extraperitoneal (Pe-TEP) approach [12]—was later developed. In Pe-TEP, the surgeon creates a preperitoneal working space directly, without entering the peritoneal cavity, by balloon or blunt dissection. This allows complete mesh placement in an extraperitoneal position while preserving peritoneal integrity.

Both ventral TAPP and Pe-TEP share the same conceptual goal: to restore the abdominal wall while keeping the mesh outside the peritoneal cavity, avoiding contact with the bowel and the need for fixation. These procedures have shown promising results, with low complication rates, less postoperative pain, and excellent functional outcomes.

The next step in this evolution was the introduction of the laparoscopic intracorporeal retromuscular anastomosis (LIRA) technique [13], which represents a refinement and functional evolution of the IPOM-Plus concept. LIRA seeks to achieve a true midline, long-lasting reconstruction without tension while preserving the advantages of a minimally invasive intraperitoneal approach. Through laparoscopic intracorporeal suturing, the medial edges of the rectus sheaths are approximated, after they have been open, to recreate the retromuscular continuity, providing an anatomical and physiological repair. This reconstruction allows correction of both primary hernias with concomitant diastasis and incisional hernia including the weak area of the previous incision, restoring the functional integrity of the abdominal wall. The midline closure is performed with a continuous suture, preferably using a barbed suture or a double-loop monofilament, which ensures even tension distribution and secure approximation of the fascial edges.

Unlike previous intraperitoneal techniques, LIRA incorporates the prosthesis as a functional substitute for the posterior rectus sheath, rather than merely a reinforcement patch. The mesh is placed intraperitoneally but acts as a neo-fascial layer, isolating the abdominal viscera and mimicking the anatomical role of the posterior sheath. This configuration reduces tension on the closure line, minimizes pain, allows a decrease of the strength of the fixation, using absorbable fixation devices, and enhances abdominal wall mechanics, while maintaining the benefits of minimal access and rapid recovery.

From a conceptual standpoint, LIRA bridges the gap between IPOM-Plus and fully retromuscular sublay repairs [14]. It preserves the simplicity, reproducibility, and shorter learning curve of intraperitoneal approaches while achieving the functional objectives of retromuscular reconstructions. Compared to eTEP or laparoscopic Rives-Stoppa techniques, LIRA requires less dissection and is more reproducible, especially in centers beginning their experience with minimally invasive abdominal wall reconstruction. This combination of anatomical logic, technical feasibility, and reduced invasiveness positions LIRA as the current evolution in laparoscopic ventral hernia repair, offering durable, tension-free, and physiologically coherent restoration of the abdominal wall [15].

However, most of the techniques that have been described until now, are indicated for hernias up to 8–10 cm. In the case of large ventral hernias, a simple intraperitoneal, retromuscular or preperitoneal repair is often insufficient to achieve complete tension-free reconstruction. For such cases, the combination of anterior component separation, which can be performed endoscopically [16], coupled with laparoscopic mesh placement with defect closure, remains a valid option allowing medial advancement of the rectus complex, although it is associated with higher rates of wound complications due to extensive subcutaneous dissection. The most popular option is, however, the posterior component separation technique with transversus abdominis muscle release (TAR) [17], which offers a more anatomical and durable reconstruction. These techniques recreate a wide retromuscular space by transecting the transverse muscle and preserving the neuromuscular bundles. However, these techniques require a high level of technical laparoscopic skills and expertise, since they involve demanding dissections.

The introduction of robotic-assisted surgery has revolutionized this field, allowing surgeons to perform with high precision what was once possible only through open surgery or by very skillful surgeons. The robotic platform provides enhanced three-dimensional visualization, superior instrument articulation, and ergonomic control, making it possible to execute eTEP and preperitoneal repairs as well as TAR procedures through a minimally invasive access. This technological advancement has expanded the indications of minimally invasive surgery to the most complex ventral and incisional hernias, combining the anatomical logic of open reconstructions with the recovery advantages of laparoscopy. As a result, robotic surgery represents the current frontier in abdominal wall reconstruction, where physiological repair, reduced morbidity, and reproducibility converge.

8.3 Lateral and Flank Hernias: Practical Diagnostic and Surgical Approach

Lateral or flank hernias often bring some of the most complex challenges in abdominal wall surgery. These defects usually lie between the costal margin and the iliac crest, lateral to the rectus sheath. Although there are some uncommon primary lumbar hernias or Spigelian hernias, most of them are developed after trauma or following retroperitoneal procedures, such as nephrectomies, aortic surgery, appendectomies, take-down ileostomy or colostomy, or bone graft harvest from the iliac crest, among others [18].

Their anatomy is variable, and every case tends to be a little different, which means that standardized solutions rarely apply. The lateral abdominal wall lacks a uniform fascial layer like the midline, consisting instead of overlapping muscular and aponeurotic structures, the external oblique, internal oblique, and transversus abdominis, each contributing to different extents along the flank, even including sometimes the anterior rectus muscles. Because of this complex architecture, these hernias often present with poorly defined margins, variable defect geometry, and limited tissue for mesh fixation.

Additionally, previous retroperitoneal dissection or infection can distort the natural planes, making identification of the preperitoneal or retromuscular space difficult. The resulting hernia sac may contain retroperitoneal fat, bowel, or kidney, and its relationship with the subcostal and iliac regions determines both the surgical access and the technical strategy. For this reason, flank hernias require individualized planning, integrating precise imaging, anatomical understanding, and a tailored operative approach to achieve durable repair while minimizing morbidity.

8.3.1 Understanding the Difference: True Hernias Versus Neuromuscular Bulges

One of the most important steps in managing a patient with a flank defect is to determine whether we are dealing with a "true fascial hernia" or a "neuromuscular or denervation bulge". The distinction is essential because the pathophysiology and treatment are completely different. A true hernia means there is a real discontinuity in the fascial layers and there's a defect through which preperitoneal fat or even bowel may protrude. Neuromuscular bulges, in contrast, come from loss of muscle tone secondary to denervation or atrophy. The fascia itself remains intact, but the wall loses its structural support [19].

From a practical point of view, the computed tomography (CT) scan is our most valuable tool. Axial and coronal views, ideally taken during Valsalva, allow us to see whether there is an actual defect in the fascia [20], while in denervation defects, the fascial layers are continuous (Figs. 8.1 and 8.2). Patients with a neuromuscular bulge should not undergo surgery; conservative measures such as physiotherapy, abdominal binders, or observation are usually best [21]. In a key study by Purnell et al. [22], who analyzed 31 postoperative flank defects, about one-third were full-thickness hernias (32%), more than half were partial defects (55%), and only 13% were pure neuromuscular bulges. These numbers remind us that while true hernias are the rule, pure denervation bulges do exist and they should be treated very differently.

8.3.2 Surgical Options for True Flank Hernias

Once it is clear that we are facing a true fascial defect, we have several minimally invasive options. The choice depends on the size, position, and previous surgical history. In general, we can consider four main strategies:

1. The retromuscular approach (eTEP or transabdominal retrorectus)

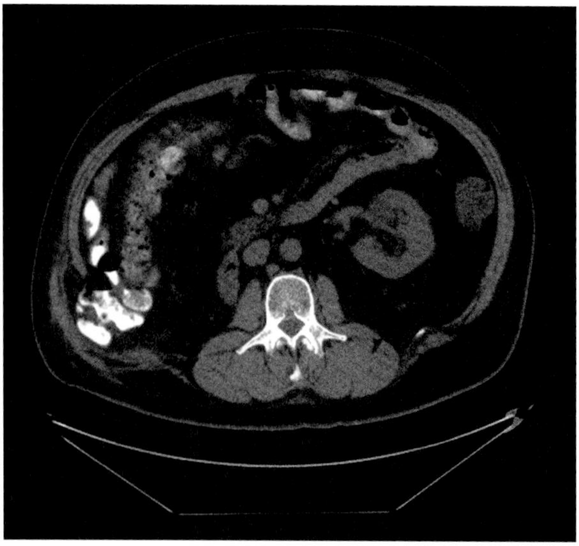

Fig. 8.1 Lateral hernia with real defect

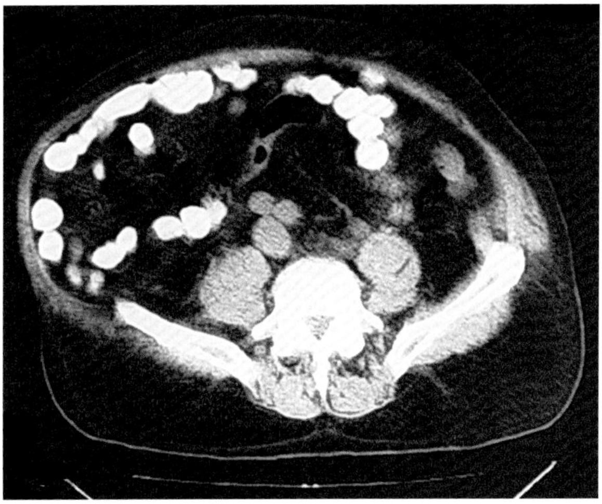

Fig. 8.2 Neuromuscular defect

2. The preperitoneal approach
3. The IPOM-Plus repair
4. The LIRA-like repair.

8.3.2.1 The Retromuscular Approach

The retromuscular plane remains one of the strongest and most durable spaces for mesh placement. Techniques such as the eTEP or transabdominal retrorectus repair allow us to reach this space laparoscopically or robotically. In lateral hernias, in order to reach this surgical plane, we have to extend this dissection laterally, performing a hemi-TAR, a unilateral transversus abdominis release, that opens the retromuscular space toward the flank [23].

This approach offers excellent mesh coverage and durable reconstruction, but it is technically demanding and requires advanced laparoscopic skills. On the other hand, we should consider that a hemi-TAR may be associated in the future with an imbalance of the abdominal wall.

8.3.2.2 The Preperitoneal Approach: The Most Logical Option

For most patients with lateral hernias, the preperitoneal laparoscopic repair is probably the most balanced and reproducible option. The lateral preperitoneal space is naturally thicker and easier to dissect than in the midline. This makes the dissection smooth and safe. Once the plane is developed, the defect is closed in the direction in which there is less tension and a large mesh is inserted, ensuring a sufficient overlap in all directions. The peritoneum is then closed over the mesh with a continuous barbed suture, isolating it from the bowel (Fig. 8.3). Regarding fixation, a self-fixing mesh or glue may be use to maintain the mesh in place. This approach offers low pain and recurrence, as well as minimal complications. In daily practice, it is the technique that fits best for most true lateral hernias.

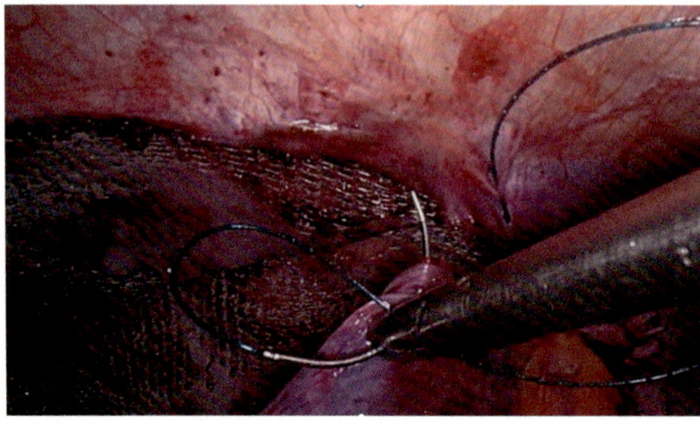

Fig. 8.3 Preperitoenal approach for a lateral/flank hernia: the peritoneum flap is closed after closing the defect and placing the mesh

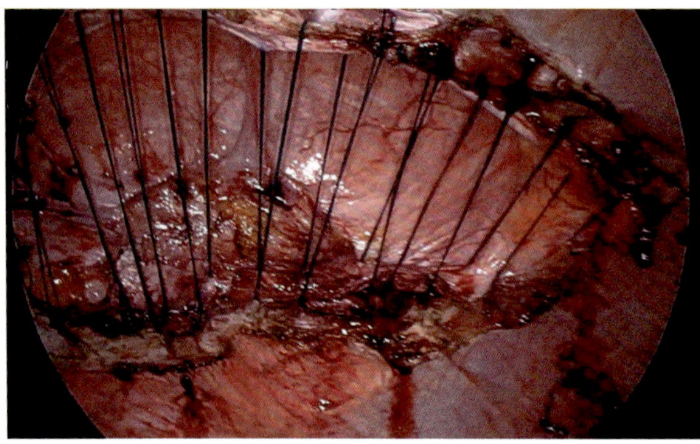

Fig. 8.4 IPOM-Plus for lateral/flank hernia: direct closure of the defect with a double-loop suture

8.3.2.3 The IPOM-Plus: Useful, but Limited

The IPOM-Plus technique (closing the defect and reinforcing it with an intraperitoneal mesh) remains a useful option when we cannot access the preperitoneal plane (Fig. 8.4). However, its success depends heavily on the defect's location. When the defect is very lateral and lies between the iliac crest and the costal margin, closure can be tricky. The space is narrow, the muscles are thin, and the defect often runs transversely. In these cases, getting a tension-free closure is difficult, and the repair can end up behaving like a bridged IPOM, with higher rates of seroma or bulging. In practice, IPOM-Plus is best reserved for small defects that are located closer to the midline, where fascial approximation is feasible and stable. Otherwise, the preperitoneal approach remains superior.

8.3.2.4 The LIRA-Like Technique: An Alternative

The LIRA-like repair extends the concept of LIRA to lateral hernias. The technique was first described by our group, who adapted the LIRA concept for the flank region through a fully intracorporeal laparoscopic approach [24]. In this method, the fascial edges are transected to decrease the tension when closing, which is performed using running sutures (barber of double-loop suture), and a mesh is placed intraperitoneally (Figs. 8.5 and 8.6). The result is a tension-free closure that preserves the

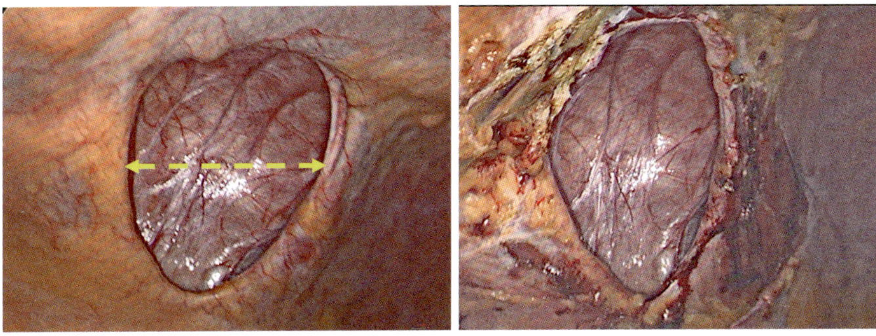

Fig. 8.5 LIRA-like technique for lateral-flank hernia: incisions are made at the lateral edge of the defect to decrease the tension when closing

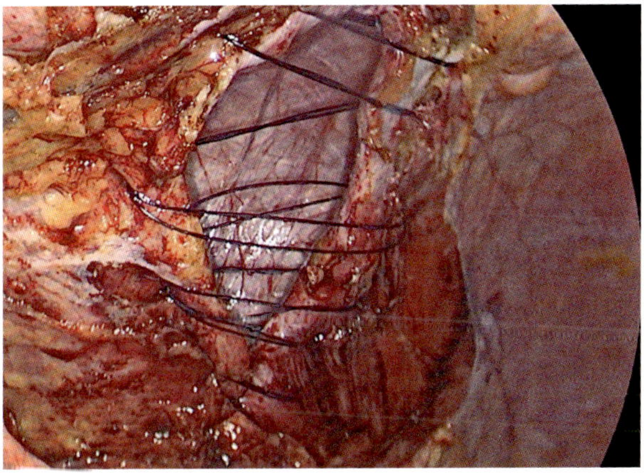

Fig. 8.6 LIRA-like technique for lateral-flank hernia: closure of the defect without tension after making incisions at the edge of the defect to decrease the tension

lateral neurovascular structures. The technique works particularly well for small-to-medium defects or when prior surgery limits preperitoneal access.

8.3.2.5 In Summary

Differentiating between true hernias and neuromuscular bulges is essential before planning surgery. Most flank defects turn out to be true hernias, but recognizing the minority of denervation bulges helps us avoid unnecessary operations. Among minimally invasive options, preperitoneal repair currently stands as the most logical and versatile approach, while the remaining techniques, retromuscular (eTEP with hemi-TAR), IPOM-Plus and LIRA-like repairs, are an alternative to the previous technique for more medial hernias.

8.4 Hernias Located Close to Bone Margins

8.4.1 Suprapubic Hernias: Practical Diagnostic and Surgical Approach

Suprapubic hernias are one of the most complex and delicate cases of the abdominal wall. They typically develop after prior lower midline incisions, prostatectomies, cystectomies, or gynecologic procedures [21]. These hernias can cause significant discomfort, pain, and cosmetic deformity. The close relationship with the bladder, iliac vessels, nerves and pubic bone adds a layer of risk that requires precise anatomical understanding and careful surgical planning.

8.4.1.1 Anatomical and Diagnostic Considerations

Below the arcuate line, the posterior rectus sheath is absent, leaving only the transversalis fascia and peritoneum to support the abdominal contents. This anatomical weakness explains why the suprapubic region is prone to herniation, especially after prior surgery. A preoperative CT scan is essential, not only to confirm the diagnosis but also to determine the precise location of the defect, its size, its relationship with the bladder, and if the hernia is below or included in the area above the arcuate line [20]. Recognizing this pattern helps guide dissection, decide the trocar location and mesh positioning during repair.

8.4.1.2 Surgical Challenges

The main challenge in repairing a suprapubic hernia lies in obtaining wide inferior overlap of the mesh over firm structures to facilitate fixing the mesh to Cooper's ligaments and pubis, in order to ensure long-term durability and minimize recurrence. However, the dissection is narrow, the tissues fragile, and the risk of bladder, vessel and nerve injury are always present.

Open sublay repairs in this area have historically been associated with high recurrence and morbidity rates owing to limited exposure and poor visualization. The development of minimally invasive techniques has significantly improved both safety and outcomes by allowing better visualization and broader mesh coverage.

8.4.1.3 Surgical Approaches

The choice of technique depends mainly on the relationship of the defect to the arcuate line and pubis and on the condition of the retromuscular or preperitoneal planes. The following order reflects the most logical and anatomical sequence of approaches:

1. Defects above the arcuate line → LIRA-TAPE (transabdominal partial extraperitoneal), eTEP repair.
2. Defects below the arcuate line → IPOM-Plus-TAPE or e-TEP repair.

Defects Above the Arcuate Line

When the defect lies above the arcuate line, the presence of a well-developed posterior rectus sheath allows for a true retromuscular reconstruction. In these cases, LIRA-like or eTEP techniques are the preferred options.

The LIRA-like approach enables the surgeon to restore the midline by reapproximating the posterior rectus sheath and closing the defect intracorporeally. A bilateral flap needs to be performed exposing the naked muscle and the arcuate line. This dissection allows one to identify not only Cooper's ligament and pubis, where the mesh could be fixed, but also all the nerves and main vessels of the pelvis. The technique is continued by opening the posterior fascia of the rectus muscle above the arcuate line. The closure is done with a continuous suture joining the rectus muscle together, below the arcuate line (Fig. 8.7), and including the medial opening of the posterior fascia above the arcuate line. Once the posterior layer is reconstructed, a mesh is placed in the retromuscular intra-abdominal position, being covered partially by the peritoneal flap performed [25] (Fig. 8.8).

The eTEP approach is equally effective, offering an extended retromuscular dissection under direct vision that continues with the access to the preperitoneal space, placing a large mesh after closing the defect.

Defects Below the Arcuate Line

When the defect lies entirely below the arcuate line, there is no posterior rectus sheath, and only the transversalis fascia and peritoneum remain to support the abdominal contents. In such cases, preperitoneal approaches are more appropriate.

The preperitoneal approach begins intraperitoneally, identifying the defect and dissecting the peritoneum and bladder from the posterior aspect of the abdominal wall. Once the defect is closed, the peritoneum is then closed over the mesh with a continuous absorbable suture, isolating it from the viscera and minimizing adhesion risk. In this approach, careful dissection of the bladder dome and prevesical fat is essential to prevent injury. The mesh must extend across the midline and laterally to both iliac vessels to ensure complete reinforcement of the suprapubic region. These minimally invasive techniques offer excellent visualization, precise control of

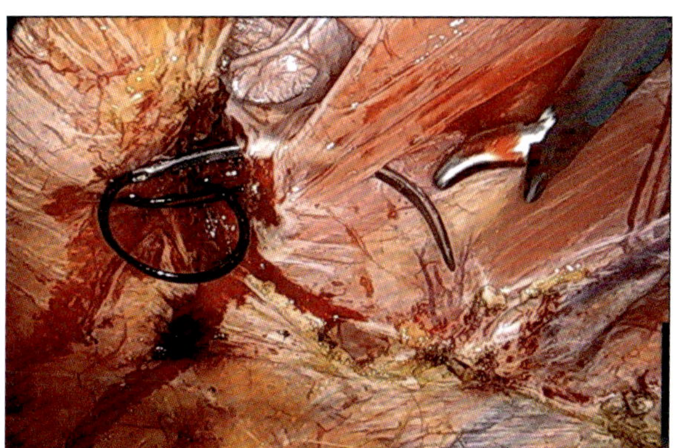

Fig. 8.7 Suprapubic hernia: closure of the rectus muscle below the arcuate line

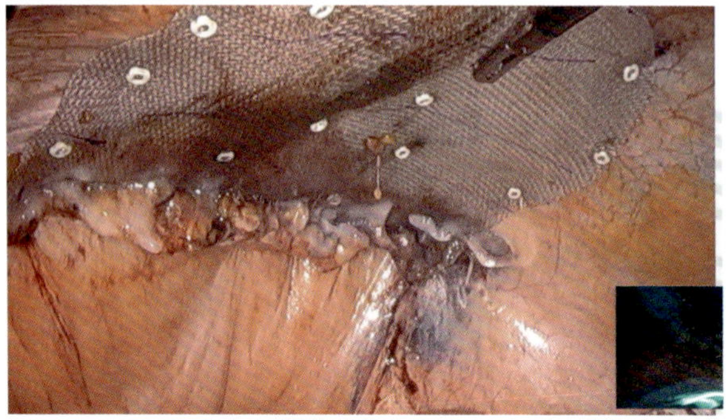

Fig. 8.8 Suprapubic hernia: the mesh is partially covered by the peritoneum (transabdominal partial extraperitoneal, TAPE)

dissection, and secure mesh positioning, with lower recurrence rates and morbidity compared with traditional open approaches.

8.4.2 Subxiphoid Hernias: Diagnostic and Laparo-Endoscopic Management

Subxiphoid hernias are among the most demanding and technically challenging abdominal wall defects. They occur just below the xiphoid process, often extending upward beneath the costal margins and downward into the upper midline. Most cases are post-sternotomy hernias following cardiac surgery, though they may also appear after previous supraumbilical incisions or reconstructions.

These defects are unique for several reasons. First, the anatomical environment is hostile: fibrotic, poorly vascularized, and lacking clear muscular planes. Second, their proximity to the diaphragm, pericardium, and costal cartilages makes dissection delicate and sometimes risky. Finally, achieving adequate mesh overlap superiorly is difficult, as the sternum and costal margins limit space for secure fixation or coverage.

Although infrequent, subxiphoid hernias can be a constant source of discomfort, chronic pain, and cosmetic deformity. For surgeons experienced in minimally invasive abdominal wall reconstruction, they represent a true test of anatomical knowledge and technical finesse.

8.4.2.1 Anatomical and Diagnostic Considerations

The subxiphoid region is a transition zone between the abdomen and the lower thorax. At the upper abdomen, the rectus sheath becomes thinner and eventually merges with the costal insertions of the diaphragm. A CT scan is indispensable before surgery. It defines the cranial extent of the defect, the presence of previous meshes or sternal wires, and whether there is any contact with the diaphragm or mediastinal structures [2]. In patients with prior cardiac surgery, it also helps rule out perigraft adhesions or aortic prostheses that could be inadvertently injured during dissection. Understanding these details is crucial for deciding whether a retromuscular or intraperitoneal repair is feasible and for planning mesh overlap.

8.4.2.2 Surgical Challenges

Several technical difficulties define the subxiphoid repair:

- Limited superior overlap: the sternum and costal cartilages restrict cranial extension of the mesh.
- Adhesions: dense fibrotic tissue from prior sternotomy or open repair obscures natural planes.
- Fixation pain: anchoring the mesh directly to the costal margin or sternum can cause chronic pain.
- Diaphragmatic risk: inadvertent injury during upper dissection can lead to pneumothorax or mediastinal communication.
- Fixation to the pericardium might lead to life-threatening conditions.

Another important aspect that complicates subxiphoid hernia repair is the morphology of the upper abdominal wall, particularly in patients with a very acute subxiphoid angle. When the costal margins converge sharply toward the midline, the available working space becomes extremely narrow, and the fascial edges cannot be approximated without significant tension. In these cases, even advanced closure techniques are limited by the geometry of the upper abdomen.

Moreover, achieving adequate cranial mesh overlap is particularly difficult when the costal angle is steep, since the upper edge of the prosthesis must conform to a concave, rigid surface. Some authors advocate leaving a small residual gap in this situation and relying on wide retromuscular reinforcement rather than forcing a high-tension closure. From a practical standpoint, when preoperative CT shows a deep subxiphoid recess or a sharply convergent costal arch, the surgeon should anticipate limited closure capacity and plan for reinforcement over reconstruction, prioritizing low tension and stable coverage over complete fascial approximation.

Because of these issues, a purely open approach often results in significant morbidity and poor exposure. Minimally invasive techniques provide better visualization, controlled dissection, and a safer environment to work near the diaphragm.

The selection of approach depends mainly on the extension of the defect and whether the upper rectus sheath and retromuscular planes are intact. The options can be summarized as follows:

- Historically, the IPOM-Plus has been the most commonly used technique for subxiphoid hernias [5]. It involves closing the fascial defect and covering it with an intraperitoneal mesh, avoiding fixation with tackers to the diaphragm, the solution being intercostal transfascial suture and glue.
- LIRA: as has been mentioned earlier, this technique looks to close the defect, as in IPOM-Plus with less tension, placing the mesh retromuscular but intraperitoneally.
- e-TEP: developing the retromuscular plane cranially toward the xiphoid and re-approximating the posterior sheath and closing the defect with barbed sutures and placing a mesh without fixation extended above the xyphoid.

- Preperitoneal approach: when the preperitoneal plane is still accessible, a laparoscopic preperitoneal repair can be attempted. The goal is to dissect the loose areolar tissue between the peritoneum and posterior fascia, extending up to the costal margins. The peritoneum is closed over the mesh to protect it from bowel contact.

8.5 Epilogue: Complex Hernias Beyond Anatomy: Reflections, and Gaps

8.5.1 Clinical Reflections

Even with the remarkable evolution of laparo-endoscopic surgery, complex ventral hernias continue to test the surgeon's understanding of anatomy, technique, and judgment. The real challenge lies in restoring both anatomy and function, while preserving the patient's quality of life. Each operation becomes a customized reconstruction rather than a standardized procedure. The surgeon must evaluate the balance between dissection extent, reconstruction stability, and biological tolerance. Preoperative imaging—especially CT with 3D reconstruction—helps plan these individualized strategies, identifying preserved tissue planes and guiding the safest approach.

8.5.2 Current Gaps in the Literature

Despite the remarkable technical evolution of laparo-endoscopic hernia surgery, the scientific literature still shows important blind spots that limit our ability to compare outcomes and refine techniques.

Equally ambiguous is the definition of complexity itself. In daily practice, "complex" does not necessarily mean "large". A small hernia located beneath the xiphoid or behind the costal arch can be far more demanding than a giant midline defect. Complexity, therefore, should be defined by the relationship of the defect to fixed anatomical structures, the condition of the surrounding tissues, and the presence of prior repairs, rather than by size alone.

In summary, the current literature reflects an extraordinary period of technical innovation but also a lack of structured scientific validation. The field has advanced faster than the evidence that supports it.

References

1. Capoccia Giovannini S, Podda M, Ribas S, et al. What defines an incisional hernia as 'complex': results from a Delphi consensus endorsed by the European Hernia Society (EHS). Br J Surg. 2024;111(1):znad346.
2. Morales-Conde S. Laparoscopic ventral hernia repair: advances and limitations. Semin Laparosc Surg. 2004;11(3):191–200.

3. Ferraro L, Formisano G, Salaj A, et al. Preliminary robotic abdominal wall reconstruction experience: single-centre outcomes of the first 150 cases. Langenbeck's Arch Surg. 2023;408(1):276.
4. LeBlanc KA, Booth WV. Laparoscopic repair of incisional abdominal hernias using expanded polytetrafluoroethylene: preliminary findings. Surg Laparosc Endosc. 1993;3(1):39–41.
5. Morales-Conde S, Cadet H, Cano A, et al. Laparoscopic ventral hernia repair without sutures – double crown technique: our experience after 140 cases with a mean follow-up of 40 months. Int Surg. 2005;90(3 Suppl):S56–62.
6. Chelala E, Thoma M, Tatete B, et al. The suturing concept for laparoscopic mesh fixation in ventral and incisional hernia repair: mid-term analysis of 400 cases. Surg Endosc. 2007;21(3):391–5.
7. Belyansky I, Daes J, Radu VG, et al. A novel approach using the enhanced-view totally extraperitoneal (eTEP) technique for laparoscopic retromuscular hernia repair. Surg Endosc. 2018;32(3):1525–32.
8. Schroeder AD, Debus ES, Schroeder M, Reinpold WM. Laparoscopic transperitoneal sublay mesh repair: a new technique for the cure of ventral and incisional hernias. Surg Endosc. 2013;27(2):648–54.
9. Schwarz J, Reinpold W, Bittner R. Endoscopic mini/less open sublay technique (EMILOS) – a new technique for ventral hernia repair. Langenbeck's Arch Surg. 2017;402(1):173–80.
10. Novitsky YW, Elliott HL, Orenstein SB, Rosen MJ. Transversus abdominis muscle release: a novel approach to posterior component separation during complex abdominal wall reconstruction. Am J Surg. 2012;204(5):709–16.
11. Maatouk M, Kbir GH, Mabrouk A, et al. Can ventral TAPP achieve favorable outcomes in minimally invasive ventral hernia repair? A systematic review and meta-analysis. Hernia. 2023;27(4):729–39.
12. Alpuche HAV, Torres FR, González JPS. Early results of eTEP access surgery with preperitoneal repair of primary midline ventral hernias and diastasis recti. A 33 patient case series of "PeTEP". Surg Endosc. 2024;38(6):3204–11.
13. Gómez-Menchero J, Guadalajara Jurado JF, Suárez Grau JM, et al. Laparoscopic intracorporeal rectus aponeuroplasty (LIRA technique): a step forward in minimally invasive abdominal wall reconstruction for ventral hernia repair (LVHR). Surg Endosc. 2018;32(8):3502–8.
14. Gómez-Menchero J, Balla A, García Moreno JL, et al. Laparoscopic intracorporeal rectus aponeuroplasty (LIRA) technique versus intraperitoneal onlay mesh (IPOM plus) for ventral hernia repair: a comparative analysis. Hernia. 2024;28(1):167–77.
15. Balthazar da Silveira CA, Rasador ACD, Marcolin P, et al. The evolving applications of laparoscopic intracorporeal rectus aponeuroplasty (LIRA) in ventral hernia repair – a systematic review. J Abdom Wall Surg. 2024,3.13497.
16. Daes J, Dennis RJ. Endoscopic subcutaneous component separation as an adjunct to abdominal wall reconstruction. Surg Endosc. 2017;31(2):872–6.
17. Balla A, Alarcón I, Morales-Conde S. Minimally invasive component separation technique for large ventral hernia: which is the best choice? A systematic literature review. Surg Endosc. 2020;34(1):14–30.
18. Moreno-Egea A, Baena EG, Calle MC, et al. Controversies in the current management of lumbar hernias. Arch Surg. 2007;142(1):82–8.
19. Salameh JR, Salloum EJ. Lumbar incisional hernias: diagnostic and management dilemma. JSLS. 2004;8(4):391–4.
20. Read JW, Ibrahim N, Jacombs ASW, et al. Imaging insights into abdominal wall function. Front Surg. 2022;9:799277.
21. Slater NJ, Montgomery A, Berrevoet F, et al. Criteria for definition of a complex abdominal wall hernia. Hernia. 2014;18(1):7–17.
22. Purnell CA, Park E, Turin SY, Dumanian GA. Postoperative flank defects, hernias, and bulges: a reliable method for repair. Plast Reconstr Surg. 2016;137(3):994–1001.

23. Hernández-Villafranca S, Qian-Zhang S, Silla IO, et al. Extended totally extraperitoneal (eTEP) treatment for lateral primary and incisional hernias. New approach to old problems. Hernia. 2022;26(6):1541–9.
24. Gómez-Valles P, Jeri-McFarlane S, Gomez-Menchero J, Morales-Conde S. Moving the concept associated to laparoscopic intracorporeal rectus aponeuroplasty (LIRA) to lateral hernia. Cir Esp (Engl Ed). 2022;100(12):780–2.
25. Jeri-McFarlane S, Gómez-Valles P, Gomez-Menchero J, et al. Expanding indication of laparoscopic intracorporeal rectus aponeuroplasty (LIRA) to suprapubic area: LIRA & TAPE. Cir Esp (Engl Ed). 2022;100(10):641–3.

Robotic Approaches for Complex Abdominal Hernias: Technical Advancements, Benefits, and Procedural Standardization

9

Giampaolo Formisano, Paolo Pietro Bianchi,
Laura Benuzzi, and Simona Giuratrabocchetta

9.1 Introduction

Surgical approaches to complex abdominal wall hernias have evolved significantly over the past decades. Traditional open repairs, while still necessary in certain cases, are often associated with extensive dissection, higher wound morbidity, and longer length of stay. The advent of laparoscopic repair reduced surgical trauma and improved recovery, yet its widespread application to large or complex hernias remains limited by restricted instrument mobility, reduced dexterity, and challenging ergonomics, particularly in the setting of distorted anatomy or dense adhesions, especially in the repair of large midline and off-midline defects because of limited mesh overlap and low rates of primary fascial closure [1, 2].

Robotic-assisted surgery offers a balance between these approaches, overcoming many of the ergonomic and technical limitations of laparoscopy while preserving the advantages of minimally invasive access and performing the same open procedure in a minimally-invasive fashion (retromuscular mesh placement with giant prosthetic reinforcement of the visceral sac combined with primary fascial closure). The robotic platform provides enhanced three-dimensional visualization, superior instrument articulation, and improved surgeon ergonomics, which facilitate advanced reconstructions [3, 4]. Compared with open surgery, robotic repair is associated with reduced wound complications, shorter length of stay, faster

G. Formisano (✉) · P. P. Bianchi
Department of Health Sciences, University of Milan, Department of General and Robotic Surgery, ASST Santi Paolo e Carlo, Milan, Italy
e-mail: giampaolo.formisano@unimi.it; paolopietro.bianchi@unimi.it

L. Benuzzi · S. Giuratrabocchetta
Department of General and Robotic Surgery, ASST Santi Paolo e Carlo, Milan, Italy
e-mail: laura.benuzzi@asst-santipaolocarlo.it;
simona.giuratrabocchetta@asst-santipaolocarlo.it

D. Cuccurullo, C. Rispoli (eds.), *Complex Abdominal Wall Surgery*, Updates in Surgery, https://doi.org/10.1007/978-3-032-24284-6_9

recovery and early return to daily activities, while offering technical versatility that extends beyond the constraints of conventional laparoscopy.

The technical advantages of robotic transversus abdominis release (TAR) include the development of posterior component separation without creation of large skin incisions and/or lipocutaneous flaps. Moreover, significant myofascial release can be achieved to aid in restoring the linea alba for larger hernia defects and to create a large space, beyond the Rives plane, for larger mesh placement.

Nevertheless, challenges remain. Robotic procedures require structured training pathways and resource allocation, and they currently involve higher direct costs compared with laparoscopic repairs. However, emerging evidence suggests that these upfront direct costs may be balanced by long-term benefits, including lower complication and recurrence rates, improved quality of life, and reduced overall healthcare utilization related to open approaches [5, 6].

This chapter focuses on robotic strategies for large midline and lateral abdominal wall hernias, emphasizing key anatomical surgical planes and technical modifications. Practical tips are provided to optimize performance, avoid common pitfalls, and enhance procedural safety and efficiency. Techniques originally developed for open abdominal wall reconstruction are described, adapted for robotic-assisted approaches to combine the benefits of minimally invasive surgery with the general principles of complex hernia repair [7, 8].

Preoperative study and planning, eventually with prehabilitation in order to control for modifiable risk factors, are fundamental. Among the most important risk factors, obesity stands out: higher BMI is consistently associated with increased wound complications, seroma formation, and recurrence [9]. Smoking is another major modifiable risk factor. The European Hernia Society (EHS) guidelines recommend smoking cessation at least 4 weeks before surgery, as smoking is strongly associated with impaired wound healing, increased infection risk, and higher recurrence rates [10], though more recent evidence suggests a possible more limited role of smoking cessation in robotic ventral hernia repair [11]. Other relevant factors include advanced age and chronic comorbidities (such as chronic obstructive pulmonary disease, hypertension, and diabetes).

Structured preoperative optimization—encompassing weight loss, smoking cessation, glycemic control, nutritional support, and treatment of comorbidities—is essential to reduce complications and improve long-term surgical success.

Preoperative imaging is strongly recommended as it plays a crucial role in surgical planning. Routine abdominal computed tomography (CT) imaging, performed both at rest and during the Valsalva maneuver, provides a precise delineation of all abdominal wall defects, assesses the integrity of the residual musculature, gives insight in terms of prior mesh positioning in the setting of recurrence and incarcerated abdominal contents, and guides operative decision-making. Prior operative reports should be reviewed in detail in case of recurrent incisional hernias. This comprehensive evaluation not only allows for tailored surgical strategies but also helps in anticipating potential intraoperative challenges.

For large defects, ultrasound is generally not preferred because of its operator dependence, limited ability to accurately measure defect size, and lack of detailed

Table 9.1 Algorithm for surgical planning and management of midline and lateral defects

	RDR > 2	**RDR > 1.5 < 2**	**RDR < 1.5**		
Midline incisional hernias	Rives repair with crossover (transabdominal or eTEP). Pure preperitoneal repair when feasible for smaller defect	Rives repair with crossover (transabdominal or eTEP), unilateral TAR may be necessary	Bilateral TAR		
	Defect <5–6 cm	**Defect >5–6 cm with at least 5 cm distance from the midline**	**Defect >5–6 cm with less than 5 cm distance from the midline**	**Defect >5–6 cm with combined midline defect (RDR > 2)**	**Defect >5–6 cm with combined midline defect (RDR < 2)**
Lateral incisional hernias	Preperitoneal repair, unilateral TAR as bailout	Unilateral TAR	Rives repair with crossover and unilateral TAR	Rives repair with crossover and unilateral TAR	Rives repair with crossover and unilateral TAR or Bilateral TAR

eTEP extended-view totally extraperitoneal, *RDR* rectus-to-defect width ratio, *TAR* transversus abdominis release

information. Magnetic resonance imaging (MRI) represents another alternative, offering even greater soft-tissue resolution compared to CT. However, MRI is not routinely used in daily practice due to its higher costs, longer acquisition times, and the fact that many surgeons may be less familiar with interpreting these images. Nevertheless, MRI can be particularly valuable in selected cases, such as recurrent hernias where a prosthetic mesh has already been placed, as it provides superior soft-tissue characterization and can help differentiate between scar tissue, mesh, and recurrent defects [12]. Ultimately, it is essential that surgeons become confident in reviewing and interpreting imaging studies for hernias, as this expertise is necessary for optimal preoperative assessment and surgical success. Personal treatment algorithm for the planning and surgical management of midline and lateral defects using robotic TAR is shown in Table 9.1.

9.2 Large Midline Incisional Hernias (Bilateral TAR)

9.2.1 Indications and Preoperative Planning

Large midline hernias often require bilateral component separation to achieve tension-free fascial closure.

There is no universally defined threshold of defect width that can be established a priori to mandate the use of posterior component separation. The indication for this technique should be individualized, taking into account patient-specific anatomical factors rather than relying on a fixed measurement. The Carbonell equation, or rectus-to-defect (RDR) width ratio, should be used to determine whether a patient is suitable for robotic TAR. According to RDR, if the sum of the width of the recti is at least twice the size of the defect, a simpler Rives repair (robotic trans-abdominal retro-muscular meshplasty [TARM], trans-abdominal retro-muscular umbilical prosthesis [TARUP] or extended-view totally extraperitoneal [eTEP] repair, according to different nomenclature and approaches) will be sufficient in most of the cases. However, if the ratio is lower than two, posterior component separation should be considered.

9.2.2 Surgical Technique

The patient is positioned supine, with the arms secured alongside the body to avoid interference with the robotic arms. Pneumoperitoneum is established using a Veress needle at Palmer's point in the left upper quadrant.

Port placement and robotic docking are critical for optimal exposure and ergonomics. A 12-mm port (Airseal®, Conmed) is positioned in the left upper quadrant. Through this port, a robotic trocar is inserted using a "trocar-in-trocar" technique. Two 8-mm robotic trocars are placed in the left flank and left iliac fossa, along the anterior axillary line, ensuring adequate distance between robotic arms and instrument mobility.

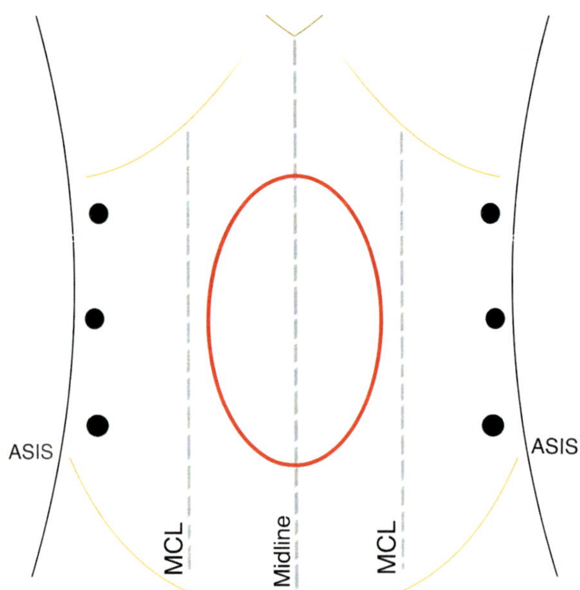

Fig. 9.1 Trocar layout for bilateral transversus abdominis release (TAR)

The assistant stands on the patient's left, and the operating table is slightly tilted in a "split-leg" position to reduce conflicts between robotic arm 1 and the patient's leg. Final trocar layout for bilateral TAR is shown in Fig. 9.1.

The robotic platform is docked from the patient's right side, with arm 1 carrying bipolar forceps, arm 2 a 30° camera, and arm 3 monopolar scissors. Retrorectus dissection is performed first contralaterally, paying attention to dissect as close to the posterior rectus sheath as possible and thus avoiding any damage to the epigastric vessels and neurovascular bundles. The retromuscular space is accessed by incising and mobilizing the posterior sheath from the overlying rectus abdominis muscle fibers. The initial incision on the posterior sheath should be performed 1–2 cm from the medial aspect of contralateral rectus muscle for adequate fascial visualization prior to anterior sheath closure. The lateral margin of the right rectus abdominis muscle and the semilunar line are then identified in a medial-to-lateral fashion, together with the neurovascular bundles that are carefully dissected and preserved to avoid rectus denervation/atrophy. Cranially, the falciform ligament is dissected free from the linea alba taking care to create a continuous flap with the posterior rectus sheath. Pure preperitoneal plane is easily developed just below the arcuate line, gaining access to Retzius and Bogros space, after dividing the transversalis fascia/attenuated posterior rectus sheath just below the junction between the arcuate line and the linea semilunaris.

TAR can subsequently be performed with different techniques and starting from different anatomical locations. It can be performed with a bottom-up approach, with a medial-to-lateral approach (Novitsky way as described in open surgery), and with a top-down approach. Anyway, bottom-up and top-down dissection will eventually join the Novitsky dissection in the mid-abdomen [7]. The simpler way to start TAR is probably the bottom-up approach in our experience, unless other incisional hernias or scar tissue related to prior abdominal wall incisions are present in that location (right lower quadrant). As a general recommendation, it is usually easier to start dissection in non-previously violated planes. It should be kept in mind, for an anatomical-based dissection, that the transversus abdominis muscle (TA) is predominantly aponeurotic in the lower part and muscular in the upper part of the abdomen, with muscular TA inserting more medially on the posterior rectus sheath and approaching the midline as we reach the subxiphoid fat pad.

Bottom-up TAR starts at the level of Bogros space with the TA muscle already in view caudally. Preperitoneal dissection is extended further laterally to create a space between the preperitoneal/pretransversalis plane and the aponeurotic TA. Bottom-up TAR can now be performed by incising the aponeurotic TA (posterior lamella of internal oblique muscle) 0.5/1 cm medially to the junction of the arcuate line with the linea semilunaris (Fig. 9.2). As we continue with our bottom-up approach, we transition to the medial-to-lateral approach as originally described by Novitsky [7]. Muscular TA becomes more evident and inserts more medially on the posterior rectus sheath in this part of the abdomen. The posterior lamella of the internal oblique muscle is then divided together with the underlying TA muscle getting access to the preperitoneal/pretransversalis plane. Paying attention not leaving any muscular structure on the "floor" of our dissection plane is of utmost importance.

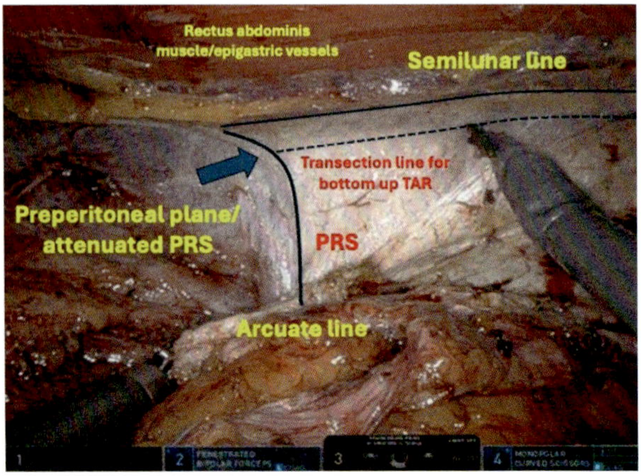

Fig. 9.2 Anatomical landmarks for bottom-up TAR. *PRS*, posterior rectus sheath; *TAR*, transversus abdominis release

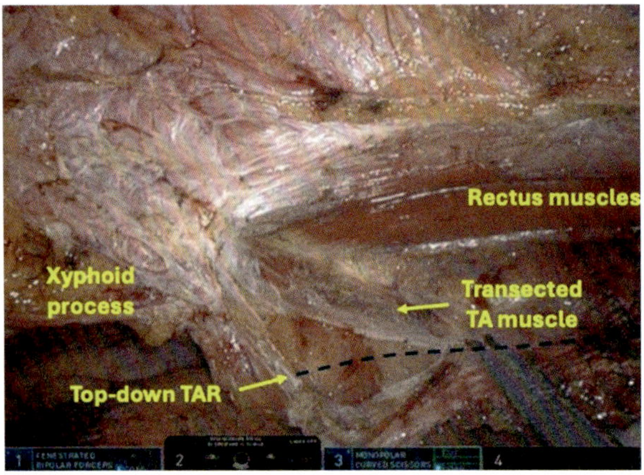

Fig. 9.3 Anatomical landmarks for top-down TAR. *TA*, transversus abdominis; *TAR*, transversus abdominis release

Lateral dissection can be performed in a pure preperitoneal plane or in a pretransversalis plane: usually, a preperitoneal plane is easily developed in the lower part of the abdomen and a transition to pretransversalis plane may be required in the mid and upper part of the dissection where the peritoneum is usually thinner and prone to multiple tears.

Top-down TAR requires adequate knowledge on the more medial insertion of TA on posterior rectus sheath at this level, as well as on preperitoneal and pretransversalis anatomy and dissection of the subxiphoid area (subxiphoid fat pad) and diaphragmatic fibers (Fig. 9.3). The posterior lamella of internal oblique and TA muscle are incised after gaining access to the preperitoneal plane below the linea alba and xiphoid process, thus exposing diaphragmatic fibers. Subxiphoid fat pad should be left in direct contact with the xiphoid process. The diaphragm interdigitates with TA and a sentinel fat pad can be identified at this level, with diaphragmatic fibers running vertically and TA fibers running horizontally (Fig. 9.4). The posterior lamella/posterior rectus sheath is then incised in a medial-to-lateral fashion, gaining access

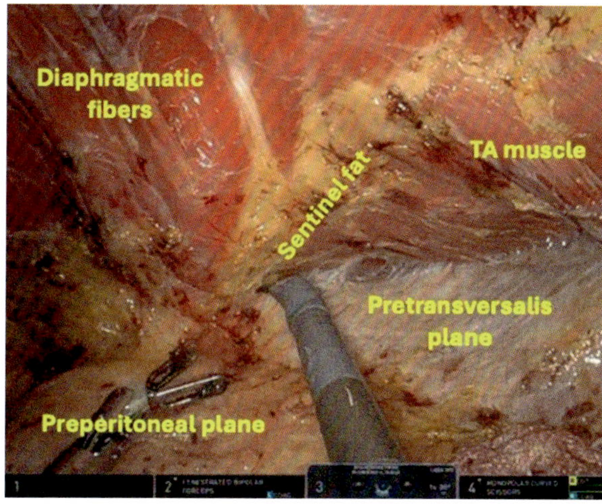

Fig. 9.4 Anatomy of subcostal area of dissection, with transversus abdominis (TA) muscle, diaphragm and sentinel fat in view

to the previously developed preperitoneal/pretransversalis plane (again, no muscle on the "floor"). A combination of bottom-up, top-down and Novitsky technique can be used according to patient- and hernia-related factors, and all the different approaches will join in the same preperitoneal plane at the end of the transection of TA.

Dissection is then continued far laterally in the preperitoneal/pretrasversalis plane to allow for larger extraperitoneal mesh overlap. Any tear at the level of the peritoneum is repaired with interrupted, running or purse-string absorbable sutures.

Three 8-mm trocars are then placed along the right anterior axillary line, the cart is de-docked and re-docked, and the same steps are performed contralaterally.

Defect closure and mesh placement complete the procedure. Posterior layer is closed with 3–0 barbed absorbable running sutured. Subsequently, hernia defect is closed with a 0 barbed absorbable running suture. Synthetic mesh (macroporous synthetic polyvinylidene fluoride [PVDF] or polypropylene mesh) is then positioned in the retromuscular/preperitoneal plane. Cyanoacrilate glue is used for mesh fixation and no sutures are used. No drain is routinely left in place.

Early series demonstrate that robotic-assisted bilateral TAR is associated with reduced postoperative pain, shorter hospital stay, and lower wound morbidity compared with traditional open bilateral TAR [13, 14].

This approach allows precise, safe, and reproducible reconstruction of large midline defects while preserving muscular function and minimizing tissue trauma, representing a significant advancement in the management of complex abdominal wall hernias.

Subdiaphragmatic dissection can be also performed in a pure preperitoneal (midline) and pretransversalis plane (off-midline) with preservation of 6–8 cm of posterior rectus sheath just caudally to the xyphoid process, in order to ensure preservation of neurovascular bundles and more stable and functional abdominal wall repair thus reducing issue related to postoperative epigastric bulging (Madrid modification of

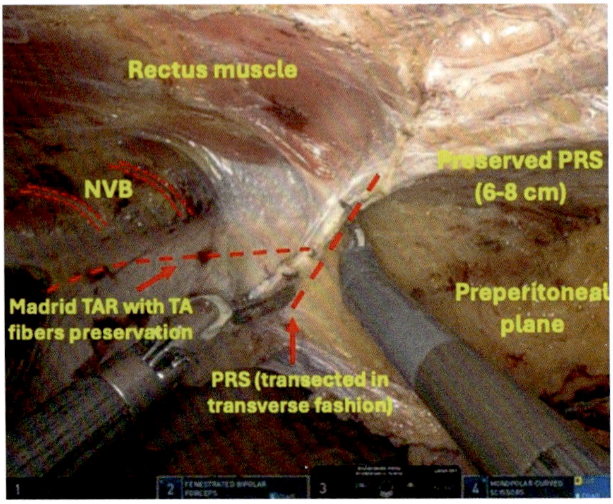

Fig. 9.5 Anatomical landmarks and TA transection line with muscular fibers preservation in TAR with Madrid modification technique. *NVB*, neurovascular bundle; *PRS*, posterior rectus sheath; *TA*, transversus abdominis; *TAR*, transversus abdominis release

TAR, as described by García-Ureña and colleagues) [8, 15]. Maintaining the integrity of the PRS also avoids injury to these diaphragmatic fibres (reducing the risks for a iatrogenic Morgagni hernia). Garcia Urena et al. have recently described a systematic dissection in ten steps that allows safe mobilization of the retromuscular plane while protecting neurovascular structures [8]. This approach is safe and effective, with favorable long-term results in complex abdominal wall reconstructions [15]. These steps can easily be performed, after proper formal training and with adequate experience in abdominal wall reconstruction, with the robotic approach (Fig. 9.5).

A single docking bottom-up approach with suprapubic port placement can be also performed for M1-M2 L1 subxiphoid, subcostal or bilateral subcostal/combined defects following the same principles of retromuscular crossover and top-down TAR (as already described) and paying attention to reach the central tendon of the diaphragm to ensure an adequate landing zone and overlap for the mesh (Fig. 9.6). In any case, according to patient and hernia-related issues, a pure preperitoneal dissection can be also performed for smaller M1-L1 incisional hernia according to the Heniford pure preperitoneal technique [16].

9.3 Lateral Incisional Hernias (Unilateral TAR)

9.3.1 Indications

Suitable candidates for unilateral TAR include large lateral incisional hernias (i.e., oostomy-site hernia or parastomal—colonic or ileal conduit hernia—with Pauli technique and bowel lateralization), possibly associated with midline incisional hernias. If RDR for the midline component is higher than two, retromuscular repair with crossover will be performed to address midline incisional hernia, together with

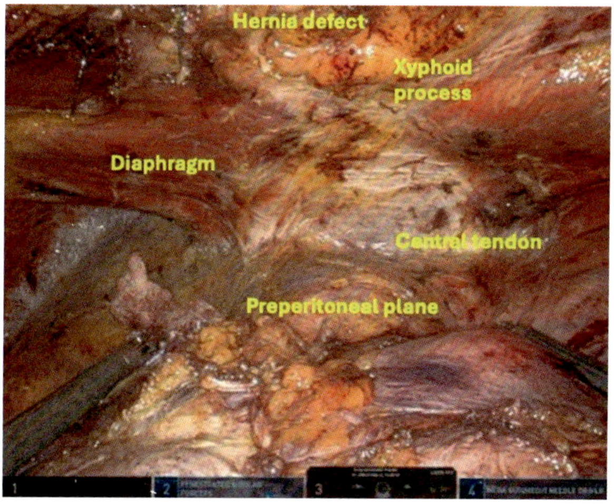

Fig. 9.6 Anatomical landmarks and final dissection after exposure of the central tendon of the diaphragm for subxiphoid defects and bottom-up approach/docking

unilateral TAR for lateral defects. In the case of lateral defects with a minimum distance from the midline less than 5 cm, retromuscular repair with crossover with a single docking approach should be performed as well to ensure adequate medial (and not only lateral) mesh overlap. Large lateral defects with at least 5 cm distance from the midline can be treated with contralateral retromuscular dissection and unilateral TAR. For smaller lateral defects (up to 4–5 cm in size), as for small suprapubic M5 and small subxiphoid M1 hernias according to the EHS classification, a pure transabdominal preperitoneal approach (rTAPP) can be performed in order to minimize the impact on patients' anatomy and abdominal wall functionality (i.e., avoid retrorectus and TAR dissection). Adequate knowledge of preperitoneal fat distribution (the so-called "fatty trident") may help in the decision-making process (Table 9.1).

9.3.2 Surgical Technique

Lateral abdominal wall hernias present unique challenges due to the involvement of the oblique and transverse muscle fibers, together with the need of adequate lateral mesh overlap to minimize the risk of recurrence. Again, it is usually easier and safer to start the dissection cranially and caudally to the fascial defect in not previously violated tissues and planes.

The patient is positioned supine, with the robot docked ipsilaterally to the fascial defect. Pneumoperitoneum is established using a Veress needle. Ports are placed contralaterally to the hernia along the anterior axillary line to allow for optimal instrument triangulation and visualization.

Surgical technique for unilateral TAR follows the same principles and surgical steps described for bilateral TAR. Care must be taken to ensure adequate lateral mesh overlap for the mesh landing zone. For lateral (or even lumbar) defects, the operating room table can be tilted or the patient can be placed in a lateral decubitus position to ensure better exposure and dissection for lateral mesh overlap. In these cases, trocars will be placed along the contralateral midclavicular line or along the midline, according to defect location. Though the key surgical steps are essentially the same, both a transabdominal approach or an eTEP approach can be used according to surgeon's preference.

9.4 Conclusions

Robotic-assisted surgery has emerged as a powerful alternative to open surgery for abdominal wall reconstruction, combining the benefits of minimally invasive access with midline functional reconstruction and retromuscular/extraperitoneal mesh placement. It may facilitate a safe and minimally invasive approach to complex midline and lateral incisional hernias with posterior component separation—TAR, with better short-term postoperative outcomes and faster recovery when compared to open surgery. Proper preoperative planning, adequate robotic training, experience in complex abdominal wall surgery and mastering abdominal wall anatomy are of paramount importance before tackling these complex procedures.

References

1. Bernardi K, Olavarria OA, Holihan JL, et al. Primary fascial closure during laparoscopic ventral hernia repair improves patient quality of life: a multicenter, blinded randomized controlled trial. Ann Surg. 2020;271(3):434–9.
2. Lindmark M, Tall J, Darkahi B, et al. Recurrence rate and mesh bulging are reduced with primary fascial closure in ventral hernia repair: the PROSECO randomized clinical trial. Br J Surg. 2025;112(9):znaf169.
3. Grossi JVM, Lee B, Belyansky I, et al. Critical view of robotic-assisted transverse abdominal release (r-TAR). Hernia. 2021;25(6):1715–25.
4. Christoffersen MW, Andresen K, Perregaard H, Henriksen NA. Robotic surgical procedures for ventral hernia repair. J Abdom Wall Surg. 2025;4:14212.
5. Awad L, Reed B, Bollen E, et al. Does robotic surgery have a role in abdominal wall reconstruction? A systematic review and meta-analysis. J Plast Reconstr Aesthet Surg. 2025;106:353–92.
6. Sabbatini F, La Regina D, Murgante Testa N, et al. Hospital costs of robotic-assisted and open treatment of large ventral hernias. Sci Rep. 2024;14(1):11523.
7. Novitsky YW, Elliott HL, Orenstein SB, Rosen MJ. Transversus abdominis muscle release: a novel approach to posterior component separation during complex abdominal wall reconstruction. Am J Surg. 2012;204(5):709–16.
8. De Luca M, López-Monclús J, Muñoz-Rodríguez JM, et al. How I do it: Madrid posterior component separation in 10 steps, with special consideration of its anatomy. Langenbeck's Arch Surg. 2024;409(1):349.
9. Nielsen KA, Tulloh B, de Beaux A, et al. Evaluation of risk factors associated with the peritoneal flap hernioplasty for complex incisional hernia repair – a retrospective review of 327 cases. Hernia. 2024;28(6):2301–9.
10. Sanders DL, Pawlak MM, Simons MP, et al. Midline incisional hernia guidelines: the European Hernia Society. Br J Surg. 2023;110(12):1732–68.

11. Kudsi OY, Kaoukabani G, Bou-Ayash N, Gokcal F. Does smoking influence the clinical outcomes of robotic ventral hernia repair? A propensity score matching analysis study. J Robot Surg. 2023;17(5):2229–36.
12. Abdelsamad A, Khalil I, Mohammed MK, et al. Conflict resolution of the beams: CT vs. MRI in recurrent hernia detection: a systematic review and meta-analysis of mesh visualization and other outcomes. Hernia. 2025;29(1):127.
13. Martin-del-Campo LA, Weltz AS, Belyansky I, Novitsky YW. Comparative analysis of perioperative outcomes of robotic versus open transversus abdominis release. Surg Endosc. 2018;32(2):840–5.
14. Bittner JG 4th, Alrefai S, Vy M, et al. Comparative analysis of open and robotic transversus abdominis release for ventral hernia repair. Surg Endosc. 2018;32(2):727–34.
15. De Luca M, Medina Pedrique M, Morejon Ruiz S, et al. The Madrid posterior component separation: an anatomical approach for effective reconstruction of complex midline hernias. J Abdom Wall Surg. 2024;3:12928.
16. Heniford BT, Ross SW, Wormer BA, et al. Preperitoneal ventral hernia repair: a decade long prospective observational study with analysis of 1023 patient outcomes. Ann Surg. 2020;271(2):364–74.

Use of Biologic, Synthetic, and Hybrid Meshes

10

Francesca Pecchini, Sofia Esposito, Vincenzo Trapani, and Micaela Piccoli

10.1 Introduction

Complex abdominal wall reconstruction is a major challenge in contemporary surgery due to its anatomical, functional, and infectious implications, requiring balance between mechanical repair, biological integration and tissue regeneration. Prosthetic materials have markedly improved outcomes in hernia recurrence and wall strength, with options ranging from permanent synthetic to fully absorbable and hybrid meshes. However, the optimal material remains controversial, especially in contaminated or high-risk fields.

Synthetic meshes are the standard in clean, elective repairs for their strength and durability, but in contaminated settings they carry higher infection risk with the need to remove the prosthesis if infected. To address this, biologic meshes were introduced to promote remodeling and host integration particularly for high-risk infection settings, though with variable long-term strength. More recently, biosynthetic materials have been developed to provide temporary scaffolds that support integration, regeneration, and neovascularization while avoiding late complications of permanent synthetics. Hybrid meshes have also recently emerged that combine synthetic scaffolds with biologic or biosynthetic components and aim to balance durability with biocompatibility.

Given the growing complexity of abdominal wall reconstruction—often involving multimorbid patients, large defects, or mesh failures—surgeons must carefully consider defect size, contamination, tissue quality, comorbidities, and surgical approach (open, laparoscopic, or robotic). This chapter provides an overview of available prosthetic materials, critically reviewing evidence and experience to

F. Pecchini (✉) · S. Esposito · V. Trapani · M. Piccoli
Division of General Surgery, Emergency and New Technologies, Baggiovara General Hospital, Modena, Italy
e-mail: francescapecc@gmail.com; esposito.sofia@aou.mo.it; trapan.vincenzo@aou.mo.it; piccoli.micaela@aou.mo.it

D. Cuccurullo, C. Rispoli (eds.), *Complex Abdominal Wall Surgery*, Updates in Surgery, https://doi.org/10.1007/978-3-032-24284-6_10

support mesh selection and offer practical recommendations for complex abdominal wall surgery.

10.2 Classification and Characteristics of Meshes

Prosthetic materials for abdominal wall reconstruction fall into four categories: synthetic, biologic, biosynthetic, and hybrid. Each has distinct properties influencing selection based on patient and surgical context. Key factors include field status (clean vs. contaminated), defect size, patient comorbidities (e.g., obesity, immunosuppression), and surgical approach (open, laparoscopic, or robotic).

10.2.1 Biologic Meshes

Biologic meshes are derived from human (allografts) or animal (xenografts) tissues—mainly dermis, pericardium, or small intestinal submucosa. They are decellularized to remove antigenic components while preserving extracellular matrix (ECM), enabling host cell infiltration, angiogenesis, and remodeling, while limiting foreign-body reaction—features useful in complex reconstruction with contamination or frailty.

Common sources:

- Porcine dermis (Strattice™, Permacol™)
- Human cadaveric dermis (AlloDerm™)
- Porcine small intestinal submucosa (Surgisis™)
- Bovine pericardium (Veritas™).

While these meshes are often used in contaminated or infected fields, their long-term mechanical strength is generally inferior to that of synthetic meshes. Moreover, their high cost remains a limiting factor for widespread use.

10.2.1.1 Mechanism of Integration and Remodeling

Biologics may be cross-linked or non-cross-linked. Cross-linking prolongs resistance to enzymatic degradation but reduces integration; non-cross-linked meshes remodel faster with better repopulation and vascularization, though at the cost of durability. Selection depends on contamination risk and need for lasting support.

10.2.1.2 Indications in Complex Settings

Typical uses include contaminated or potentially infected fields (classified by Centers for Disease Control [CDC] as a clean-contaminated or contaminated wound, CDC II–IV [1], and by the Ventral Hernia Working Group as VHWG grade 3–4 [2]), large hernias with tenuous closure, fistula-associated reconstruction, and high-risk hosts (immunocompromised, oncologic). When feasible, reinforcement after primary closure is preferred over true bridging.

10.2.1.3 Clinical Outcomes and Limitations

Recent randomized controlled trials have provided strong evidence regarding biologic meshes in complex abdominal wall reconstruction. Rosen et al. showed in a multicenter randomized trial on contaminated ventral hernias that recurrence was significantly lower with synthetic mesh (5.6%) compared to biologic mesh (20.5%), without differences in serious adverse events [3]. Similarly, Olavarría et al. reported higher complication rates in the biologic group (42.4% vs. 21.6%) [4]. The PRICE trial by Harris et al. also demonstrated no clinical advantage for biologic mesh in clean or contaminated fields [5], with suboptimal long-term outcomes and high costs compared with synthetic meshes [6].

These observations are consistent with several non-randomized series, which generally reported comparable rates of surgical site occurrences, surgical site infections, and hernia recurrence between biologic and synthetic prostheses [7–9]. However, the interpretation of these findings is limited by substantial heterogeneity in patient selection, defect size, closure strategies, and duration of follow-up.

In general, two consistent caveats emerge in complex reconstruction: (i) bridging with biologic mesh carries higher recurrence than reinforcement after primary fascial approximation; and (ii) long-term durability of biologics is generally inferior to permanent synthetics, with outcomes modulated by source tissue and cross-linking. Given the substantially higher cost, most contemporary practice limits biologics to selected high-risk or contaminated scenarios where permanent synthetics are contraindicated or judged unsafe (pending patient- and defect-specific considerations).

10.2.1.4 Cost Considerations

Cost-effectiveness remains unclear. Without outcome advantages and given higher prices, their use should be restricted to carefully selected patients where infection risk may offset costs, ideally within institutional pathways.

10.2.2 Synthetic Meshes

Synthetic meshes, composed of non-biological polymers, remain the most reliable option for clean and selected contaminated fields, providing durable reinforcement, lower recurrence, and favorable cost-effectiveness compared with biologics [3–7, 10]. Cost-effectiveness analyses have consistently favored synthetic meshes over biologics in complex abdominal wall reconstruction [7].

Their use in complex reconstruction must balance long-term support with risks of infection, erosion, and pain.

10.2.2.1 Types and Materials

Common materials include:

- Polypropylene (PP): widely adopted due to its strength, flexibility, and cost-effectiveness.

- Expanded polytetrafluoroethylene (ePTFE): known for low tissue ingrowth and minimal adhesion, often used in intraperitoneal applications.
- Polyethylene terephthalate (PET): historically used, less common today due to higher infection and erosion rates.
- Polyvinylidene fluoride (PVDF): offers good biostability and minimal inflammatory response.

Meshes may be permanent or partially absorbable, and classified by weight (light vs. heavy), porosity (macro vs. micro), and filament structure (mono- vs. multifilament).

Design variables that influence outcomes in complex cases are:

- Weight & porosity: lightweight, macroporous (≥~1 mm or >75 μm pore size) meshes favor tissue ingrowth and reduce chronic foreign-body reaction thus reducing infection risk compared with heavy, microporous constructs.
- Monofilament vs. multifilament: monofilament macroporous meshes are generally preferred to limit bacterial harboring.
- Barrier/composite designs for intraperitoneal placement (intraperitoneal onlay mesh, IPOM) aim to reduce visceral adhesions while maintaining parietal ingrowth.

10.2.2.2 Positioning and Fixation

Retrorectus/sublay reinforcement after fascial closure is preferred for durability and fewer complications. Onlay and IPOM remain options in reoperations or limited component separation. Fixation may use sutures, tacks, or both. In hostile fields, meticulous debridement, dead-space control, and thoughtful drain strategy are pivotal regardless of mesh type.

10.2.2.3 Complications

Complications include surgical site infections (SSI) and surgical site occurrences (SSO), seroma, fistula, mesh erosion, and pain. Risks are higher with microporous, heavyweight, multifilament, or bridging repairs. Patient comorbidities and contamination level strongly affect outcomes.

10.2.2.4 Contamination Spectrum

In clean or clean-contaminated fields, permanent synthetics remain first-line. In contaminated/dirty settings (CDC II–IV; VHWG 3–4), extraperitoneal placement may be feasible after adequate source control. Biosynthetic or long-term absorbables are alternatives when permanent material is undesirable.

10.2.2.5 Biosynthetic Versus Synthetic in Complex Abdomen

Non-randomized studies comparing biosynthetic (long-term absorbable) and permanent synthetic meshes in contaminated or high-risk incisional hernia repairs report no consistent superiority of one approach across core outcomes:

- Recurrence: generally comparable between biosynthetic and synthetic groups.
- SSI/SSO: similar rates overall; differences, when present, are study- and context-dependent.
- Mesh removal/explant: typically low and comparable; decisions are often driven by deep infection or enteric fistula rather than mesh class per se.

These conclusions are supported by many authors, which collectively suggest that biosynthetics can serve as a reasonable alternative to permanent synthetics in selected contaminated complex reconstructions, particularly when surgeons aim to limit permanent foreign material [11–14]. However, the observational design, heterogeneous case mix, and variable follow-up limit definitive inferences. Longer-term durability of biosynthetics beyond the absorption window remains a key question.

10.2.2.6 Practical Takeaways

- Prioritize primary fascial closure + extraperitoneal reinforcement with a mesh whenever achievable.
- Reserve bridging for non-closable defects and counsel regarding higher recurrence regardless of material.
- In contaminated fields with good source control, carefully selected permanent synthetics may be acceptable; biosynthetic meshes are a viable alternative when minimizing permanent foreign body is a priority, recognizing the evidence is observational.
- Standardize perioperative protocols (decontamination, negative pressure wound therapy [NPWT] where appropriate) to modulate risk more than mesh class alone.

10.2.3 Biosynthetic Meshes

Biosynthetic meshes are fully synthetic but composed of absorbable polymers such as poly-4-hydroxybutyrate (P4HB, Phasix™) or polyglycolide-trimethylene carbonate (PGA:TMC, Gore Bio-A™). They provide temporary reinforcement during healing, then resorb and are replaced by vascularized host tissue. Compared with permanent synthetics, they may induce less chronic inflammation and foreign-body reaction.

The most commonly used:

- Poly-4-hydroxybutyrate (P4HB, Phasix™): long-term, 18 months, absorbable polymer with gradual resorption, leaving behind host tissue reinforcement.
- Polyglycolide-trimethylene carbonate (PGA:TMC, Gore Bio-A™): a 3D open-pore scaffold promoting cellular infiltration, neovascularization, and remodeling, with complete resorption in 6–7 months.

10.2.3.1 Clinical Evidence and Outcomes

The clinical use of biosynthetic meshes in complex abdominal wall reconstruction has been investigated primarily through observational studies. Parker et al. reported that P4HB mesh was associated with low rates of surgical site occurrences and acceptable recurrence when used in contaminated ventral hernias, suggesting that biosynthetics may represent a safe alternative in challenging scenarios [11]. Similarly, Sahoo et al. observed that biosynthetic meshes achieved lower recurrence rates compared with biologic prostheses in contaminated fields, supporting their use when permanent synthetics are contraindicated [12].

Specific evidence for PGA:TMC comes from the multicenter prospective COBRA study, which evaluated Gore Bio-A™ in 104 patients with clean-contaminated or contaminated ventral hernia repair [15]. At 24 months, hernia recurrence was 17% overall (14% when considering only midline recurrence), with no cases of complete mesh explantation despite an 18% rate of SSI. Importantly, retrorectus placement was associated with lower recurrence compared to intraperitoneal positioning, and quality of life scores (EuroQol-5 Dimensions [EQ-5D] and Short Form [SF-12]) significantly improved over time.

Taken together, these findings suggest that biosynthetic meshes may provide a compromise between the durability of synthetics and the biocompatibility of biologics, although the current evidence is limited by the predominance of non-randomized designs and relatively short follow-up. Early clinical reports, summarized by Morales-Conde et al. [16], indicate that bioresorbable meshes could be considered an alternative to synthetic and biologic mesh reinforcement in grade 2–3 ventral hernia repair settings, although long-term randomized data are still lacking.

10.2.3.2 Limitations and Cost Considerations

Evidence remains limited, with short follow-up and non-randomized designs. Biosynthetics are costlier than synthetics but generally cheaper than biologics, raising interest in their cost-effectiveness. Rognoni et al. estimated that their progressive adoption in complex ventral hernia repair could lead to substantial cost savings for the healthcare system, while maintaining acceptable safety [17]. In a multicenter registry, the same group reported mid-term outcomes with Phasix™ and Phasix ST™ in VHWG 2–3 patients, showing low recurrence (8% at 36 months), rare mesh explantation for infection (1.3%), and sustained improvements in quality of life [18].

In summary, biosynthetic meshes—including P4HB and PGA:TMC—have emerged as promising options for complex abdominal wall reconstruction, particularly in high-risk or contaminated fields where biologic and permanent synthetic meshes show important limitations.

10.2.4 Hybrid Meshes

Hybrid meshes are an evolving category for complex abdominal wall reconstruction, combining synthetic strength with biologic or biosynthetic elements to enhance tissue integration, vascularization, and resistance to infection. Their rationale is to merge the durability of synthetics with the remodeling capacity of biologics, making them attractive in contaminated or high-risk fields where synthetics alone may be unsafe and biologics insufficient. These materials are designed for potential use also in contaminated or high-risk settings where synthetic meshes may be contraindicated, but where greater mechanical strength is desired than that offered by biologics alone. Clinical data remain limited, but early results are encouraging in selected patient populations.

10.2.4.1 Definition and Composition

Hybrid constructs typically integrate:

- Permanent synthetics (e.g., polypropylene, PTFE)
- Biosynthetic polymers (e.g., P4HB, PGA:TMC) or biologic ECM collagen (porcine/bovine).

This design aims to ensure strength, improve host integration, reduce foreign-body response, and enhance performance in challenging environments.

10.2.4.2 Current Products

- Synecor™: PGA:TMC scaffold for vascularization, PTFE fibers for permanent strength, and optional PGA:TMC film to reduce adhesions.
- Ovitex™: polymer fibers interwoven with ovine ECM collagen.
- Zenapro™: synthetic scaffold reinforced with porcine dermal matrix.

Despite design differences, all seek a synthetic-biologic synergy for durability and tolerance.

10.2.4.3 Clinical Evidence

Data are limited to observational series and registries. Early results show feasibility in contaminated hernia repairs, with SSI and recurrence rates similar to synthetics, improved integration compared with biologics, and occasional lower explant rates. Recurrence remains variable and strongly influenced by closure strategy. No randomized trials or long-term data exist, leaving durability and cost-effectiveness unproven.

10.2.4.4 Limitations

High cost, though less than biologics, and selection bias in published studies restrict broader adoption.

10.3 Clinical Decision-Making and Mesh Selection

International guidelines support individualized mesh selection in complex abdominal wall repair, guided by three main factors: surgical field status, patient comorbidities, and feasibility of fascial closure.

In clean cases in low risk patients, permanent synthetic meshes remain standard, offering durability, low recurrence, and cost-effectiveness. Lightweight macroporous synthetics placed extraperitoneally yield optimal results.

In high risk patients or in contaminated fields (CDC II–III; VHWG 3), permanent synthetics can still be safe if closure and source control are achieved. When concern exists over permanent implants, biosynthetics offer temporary reinforcement, with evidence showing outcomes comparable to synthetics, though long-term durability remains uncertain.

In dirty fields (CDC IV; VHWG 4), delayed repair is preferred; if immediate reconstruction is required, biologics may be used as reinforcement but not for bridging due to high recurrence.

Patient factors such as obesity, diabetes, immunosuppression, or prior mesh infection should further influence choice. In such settings, biologic or biosynthetic alternatives may be preferable despite limited evidence.

Technical strategy often outweighs material choice: tension-free fascial closure, component separation, meticulous tissue handling, and adjuncts like negative pressure therapy are key to success.

In summary, mesh selection depends on aligning material with patient and field (see Fig. 10.1). Synthetics remain first-line in clean repairs, biosynthetics are a valuable alternative in selected contaminated scenarios, and biologics retain a niche role in high-risk, complex cases.

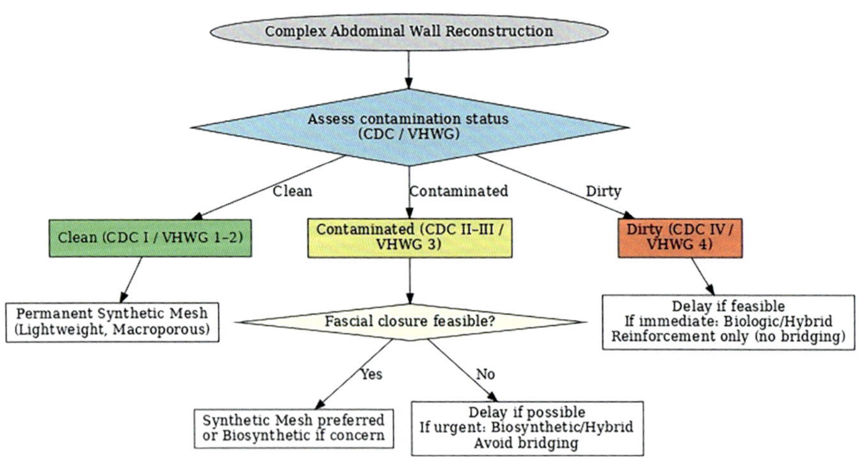

Fig. 10.1 Flowchart for mesh selection in complex abdominal wall reconstruction. *CDC*, Centers for Disease Control; *VHWG*, Ventral Hernia Working Group

10.4 Special Considerations

Economic and quality of life aspects are central in complex abdominal wall repair. A PRICE trial sub-analysis showed biologics are more costly without quality of life benefit over synthetics [9]. Harris et al. confirmed synthetics prevent recurrences more effectively and remain economically sustainable [3].

10.4.1 Reoperations and Recurrences

Recurrent hernias and reoperations represent one of the most challenging scenarios in complex abdominal wall surgery. Previous mesh placement, adhesions, and compromised tissue quality often restrict available reconstructive options. Permanent synthetics remain effective when placed in an extraperitoneal position after careful adhesiolysis and debridement, but risk of enteric injury and infection is increased. In these settings, biosynthetic or hybrid meshes may be considered, particularly when previous infection or intolerance to permanent materials has occurred.

10.4.2 Immunosuppressed and Oncologic Patients

Patients undergoing immunosuppressive therapy or with active malignancy present impaired wound healing and a higher susceptibility to infection. Evidence is limited, but caution is advised with permanent synthetics. Biologic or biosynthetic meshes may offer better tolerance, though recurrence remains elevated. Close monitoring and multidisciplinary input are recommended.

10.4.3 Contaminated Redo Surgery

In septic reoperations (e.g., mesh infection, fistula takedown), explantation is often required. Reconstruction depends on residual wall quality and contamination. Biologic or biosynthetic meshes may serve as temporary reinforcement, but delayed definitive repair is preferable when feasible.

10.5 Economic and Availability Considerations

Cost remains a critical factor in the selection of prosthetic material for complex cases. Permanent synthetic meshes are the most cost-effective, supported by strong evidence in clean cases and selected contaminated repairs. Biologic are considerably more expensive, with limited evidence of superiority, restricting their use to niche indications, while biosynthetics occupy an intermediate position in terms of cost and may represent a pragmatic compromise in settings where avoidance of permanent foreign material is desirable. Institutional availability, reimbursement policies, and resource allocation therefore influence real-world practice as much as clinical evidence.

10.6 Conclusions

Complex abdominal wall reconstruction is evolving with new prosthetic materials. No mesh is universally ideal; optimal outcomes depend on aligning mesh type with patient, defect, and surgical field. Synthetic meshes remain the standard in clean and selected contaminated cases, offering durability, low recurrence, and best cost-effectiveness. Biologics, despite theoretical advantages, should be limited to highly selected or dirty fields, avoiding bridging due to poor durability and high cost. Biosynthetics provide temporary yet robust scaffolds, bridging the gap between biologics and synthetics; early data are encouraging but long-term randomized trials are needed. Hybrid meshes aim to combine strength with biological integration, with preliminary but promising results.

Mesh selection must consider comorbidities, defect features, and contamination, balancing durability, infection risk, and cost. Technical execution is often more decisive than mesh type: tension-free closure, using component separation when required, source control, and adjuncts such as NPWT remain critical.

Future research should deliver high-quality randomized controlled trials comparing all mesh categories in well-defined complex settings. Until then, individualized decision-making, integrating current evidence, surgical expertise, and institutional resources, is essential.

In summary, the guiding principle remains: the right mesh, for the right patient, in the right field.

References

1. Mangram A, Horan T, Pearson M, et al. Guideline for prevention of surgical site infection, 1999. Centers for Disease Control and Prevention (CDC) Hospital Infection Control Practices Advisory Committee. Am J Infect Control. 1999;27(2):97–132.
2. Ventral Hernia Working Group, Breuing K, Butler CE, et al. Incisional ventral hernias: review of the literature and recommendations regarding the grading and technique of repair. Surgery. 2010;148(3):544–58.
3. Rosen MJ, Krpata DM, Petro CC, et al. Biologic vs synthetic mesh for single-stage repair of contaminated ventral hernias: a randomized clinical trial. JAMA Surg. 2022;157(4):293–301.
4. Olavarria OA, Bernardi K, Dhanani NH, et al. Synthetic versus biologic mesh for complex open ventral hernia repair: a pilot randomized controlled trial. Surg Infect. 2021;22(5):496–503.
5. Harris HW, Primus F, Young C, et al. Preventing recurrence in clean and contaminated hernias using biologic versus synthetic mesh in ventral hernia repair: the PRICE randomized clinical trial. Ann Surg. 2021;273(4):648–55.
6. Majumder A, Winder JS, Wen Y, et al. Comparative analysis of biologic versus synthetic mesh outcomes in contaminated hernia repairs. Surgery. 2016;160(4):828–38.
7. Herrero A, Gonot Gaschard M, Bouyabrine H, et al. Comparative study of biological versus synthetic prostheses in the treatment of ventral hernias classified as grade II/III by the Ventral Hernia Working Group. J Visc Surg. 2022;159(2):98–107.

8. Chamieh J, Tan WH, Ramirez R, et al. Synthetic versus biologic mesh in single-stage repair of complex abdominal wall defects in a contaminated field. Surg Infect. 2017;18(2):112–8.
9. Shao JM, Ayuso SA, Deerenberg EB, et al. Biologic mesh is non-inferior to synthetic mesh in CDC class 1 & 2 open abdominal wall reconstruction. Am J Surg. 2022;223(2):375–9.
10. Diab MM, Patel S, Young C, et al. Quality of life measures and cost analysis of biologic versus synthetic mesh for ventral hernia repair: the preventing recurrence in clean and contaminated hernias randomized clinical trial. Surgery. 2024;175(4):1063–70.
11. Parker MJ, Kim RC, Barrio M, et al. A novel biosynthetic scaffold mesh reinforcement affords the lowest hernia recurrence in the highest-risk patients. Surg Endosc. 2021;35(9):5173–8.
12. Sahoo S, Haskins IN, Huang LC, et al. Early wound morbidity after open ventral hernia repair with biosynthetic or polypropylene mesh. J Am Coll Surg. 2017;225(4):472–480e1.
13. Keogh K, Slater K. Comparison of biosynthetic versus synthetic mesh in clean and contaminated ventral hernia repairs. ANZ J Surg. 2020;90(4):542–6.
14. Morrison BG, Gledhill K, Plymale MA, et al. Comparative long-term effectiveness between ventral hernia repairs with biosynthetic and synthetic mesh. Surg Endosc. 2023;37(8):6044–50.
15. Rosen MJ, Bauer JJ, Harmaty M, et al. Multicenter, prospective, longitudinal study of the recurrence, surgical site infection, and quality of life after contaminated ventral hernia repair using biosynthetic absorbable mesh: the COBRA study. Ann Surg. 2017;265(1):205–11.
16. Morales-Conde S, Hernández-Granados P, Tallón-Aguilar L, et al. Ventral hernia repair in high-risk patients and contaminated fields using a single mesh: proportional meta-analysis. Hernia. 2022;26(6):1459–71.
17. Rognoni C, Bassi UA, Cataldo M, et al. Budget impact analysis of a biosynthetic mesh for incisional hernia repair. Clin Ther. 2018;40(11):1830–1844.e4.
18. Rognoni C, Cuccurullo D, Borsoi L, et al. Clinical outcomes and quality of life associated with the use of a biosynthetic mesh for complex ventral hernia repair: analysis of the "Italian Hernia Club" registry. Sci Rep. 2020;10(1):10706.

Management of Parastomal Hernias: Challenges and Innovative Solutions

11

McKell Quattrone and Eric M. Pauli

11.1 Introduction

Parastomal hernias are common following stoma formation, occurring in up to 28–58% of ileostomies and colostomies respectively [1, 2], with an increasing number of parastomal hernia repairs annually [3]. They are associated with patient morbidity ranging from minor skin complications related to leakage and pouching issues to bowel obstruction and ischemia related to incarcerated and strangulated bowel [4, 5]. Parastomal hernias additionally pose a complex management challenge due to the need for an ongoing fascial defect at the repair site to accommodate the stoma bowel. This inherent risk of recurrence from the ongoing fascial defect plus the risk of infectious and stoma-related complications adds to the complexity of these repairs and makes consensus for management recommendations challenging.

11.2 Preoperative Planning and Considerations

No definitive management recommendations exist for the surgical management of parastomal hernias based upon the most recent European Hernia Society (EHS) and the American Society of Colon and Rectal Surgeons' clinical practice guidelines. This is largely due to a lack of comparative high-quality evidence between repair techniques [6, 7], further highlighting the complexity in the clinical and surgical management of these patients. As such, the clinical and surgical management of parastomal hernias largely remains at the operating surgeon's discretion based upon personal expertise and clinical judgement. Preoperative cross-sectional imaging is recommended to evaluate hernia characteristics and guide operative decision

M. Quattrone · E. M. Pauli (✉)
Division of Minimally Invasive and Bariatric Surgery, Penn State Health Milton S. Hershey Medical Center, Hershey, PA, USA
e-mail: mquattrone@pennstatehealth.psu.edu; epauli@pennstatehealth.psu.edu

D. Cuccurullo, C. Rispoli (eds.), *Complex Abdominal Wall Surgery*, Updates in Surgery, https://doi.org/10.1007/978-3-032-24284-6_11

making [6]. The EHS classification system provides information to characterize parastomal hernias based upon size (≤5 cm or >5 cm), presence of a midline defect and if the hernia is recurrent. However, no current management recommendations exist based upon classification.

In asymptomatic patients or in patients who can manage their symptoms without significant impact to quality of life, a watchful waiting approach is recommended due to the high risk of recurrence following repair. This is particularly the case in patients with significant comorbidities where surgical risk may be prohibitive. Watchful waiting has been shown to be safe, with only a small percentage of patients requiring emergency operation for obstruction [8]. This approach should be tailored to individual patients, however, as patients with a high hernia sac to neck ratio or symptomatic patients with a history of obstruction may be at higher risk of progression to emergency surgery.

In patients with intolerable hernia symptoms (most notably pain or peristomal skin complications) without concern for obstruction or strangulation necessitating urgent intervention, efforts for patient optimization should be undertaken. Patient factors including BMI, smoking status, diabetes, inflammatory bowel disease (IBD) status and immunosuppressive medications should be considered in the perioperative decision making and optimized as able. Patients who are active smokers should be counselled on smoking cessation and patients with morbid obesity should undergo weight loss prior to repair. Additionally, all patients should be up to date on age-appropriate screening endoscopy recommendations. All patients with malignancy as the indication for their stoma creation should have ideally completed any adjuvant treatment and have remained disease free on up-to-date imaging and endoscopic surveillance.

The patient's past surgical history should be reviewed, noting all prior abdominal operations, the type of stoma (colostomy vs. ileostomy, loop vs. end), any prior hernia repairs, and if an associated midline hernia defect is also present. Patients should finally be evaluated by a colorectal surgeon to determine if they are a candidate for stoma reversal prior to repair, as this is associated with a lower recurrence rate than if the stoma is not reversed [9]. If the stoma can be reversed, the hernia defect can be repaired as an incisional hernia at the time of the reversal procedure.

11.3 Surgical Repair Techniques

Multiple different parastomal repair techniques exist with respect to operative approach, stoma management, mesh location, mesh configuration and mesh type. Surgical repair of parastomal hernias can largely be broken down based on the following components:

1. Operative approach: midline laparotomy, peristomal, minimally invasive (laparoscopic vs. robotic)
2. Primary repair vs. mesh-based repair
3. Mesh location: onlay vs. sublay (preperitoneal or retromuscular) vs. underlay.

If stoma reversal is not feasible or indicated, consideration should be given to the intraoperative management of the stoma itself, including whether the stoma requires local revision, relocation to a separate site, or can be left *in situ*, as this may impact the repair type and mesh configuration selected.

11.3.1 Mesh Configuration

The need for an ongoing *in situ* stoma poses some unique considerations for mesh-based repairs. Numerous configurations have been described for placing mesh around the stoma bowel, including a keyhole, cruciate and Sugarbaker configuration. The keyhole mesh configuration involves cutting a slit from the mesh edge with a circular or cruciate defect in the mesh center to accommodate the *in situ* stoma bowel. The cut edge of the mesh can then be reapproximated with permanent suture. A cruciate configuration, in contrast, involves creating an X-shaped defect in the center of the mesh for the stoma bowel to be delivered through. Use of this configuration involves taking down the stoma at the mucocutaneous junction to allow for passage of the bowel through the mesh and reforming the stoma. Recurrences with use of these configurations are often due to the enlargement of the mesh defects over time.

In a Sugarbaker configuration, no defects are cut within the mesh. Instead, the mesh is placed flat like a sling against the stoma bowel. This creates a tunnel for the bowel and creates lateralization of the bowel to the abdominal wall until it reaches the mesh edge. While initially used in the underlay position (intraperitoneal), it can additionally be used for sublay (retromuscular repairs). Studies have found that modified Sugarbaker configurations have lower recurrence rates compared to keyhole repairs [10], particularly with laparoscopic underlay repairs. A variety of other configuration techniques have been described in the literature, including a funnel-shaped mesh and the sandwich technique, which involves a combination of keyhole and Sugarbaker mesh, without improvements in outcomes.

11.3.2 Mesh Selection

No consensus exists for mesh selection for parastomal hernia management without any demonstrated benefit between mesh types. Mesh selection is largely based on personal preference and individual operative and patient characteristics. Special consideration again should be given to the close proximity of mesh to stoma bowel due to the potential risk of mesh infection and mesh erosion. Because of this, a light or medium weight synthetic mesh is often preferred to a heavy-weight mesh. No benefit has been demonstrated regarding recurrence rates or mesh-related complications with the use of biologic mesh. Additionally, if mesh is placed in an intraperitoneal position, coated mesh should be used to face the abdominal cavity.

11.3.3 Primary Repairs

Primary repairs should be avoided if a mesh-based repair is feasible due to the high risk of recurrence. They are a suitable option for emergent cases where there is concern for bowel compromise, significant contamination or in complex patients who are not candidates for a larger mesh-based repair. However, they are associated with an over 50% recurrence rate, with some literature noting a 100% recurrence rate over time. These repairs can be approached through either a local peristomal incision or a midline laparotomy. Peristomal incisions allow for a local repair and reduction of the hernia contents without more extensive exploration. If a larger intra-abdominal exploration is necessary, a midline laparotomy can be utilized. In all cases, preoperative imaging should be reviewed to evaluate the location of the hernia contents and hernia sac in relation to the hernia defect.

If a peristomal incision is used, a curvilinear incision should be made approximately 10 cm from the stoma site, corresponding to the site of hernia sac on imaging. Dissection can then be carried down to the anterior fascia and the stoma can be circumferentially mobilized from the hernia sac and surrounding tissue. If there is noted to be redundancy of the bowel within the subcutaneous tissue, a local stoma revision can be performed. Once the fascia edges are circumferentially freed, it can be closed with slowly absorbable monofilament suture.

As an alternative to monofilament suture, mesh-suture (Duramesh®, Mesh Suture Inc, Chicago, IL) can additionally be used for defect closure. Its composition of multiple polypropylene strands to create a macroporous mesh scaffold helps to aid in repair strength, reduce suture pull-through and increase in tissue incorporation compared to monofilament suture (Fig. 11.1). It has been shown to be safe for the management of parastomal hernias with low short-term complication and recurrence rates [11]; however, long-term study is needed.

Regardless of suture type, a figure-of-eight closure technique is often preferred for the repair. Care should be taken to close the defect by taking strong bites of anterior fascia while avoiding injury to the stoma bowel and ensuring the closure is not too tight to cause a luminal obstruction or alter blood supply to the stoma. While

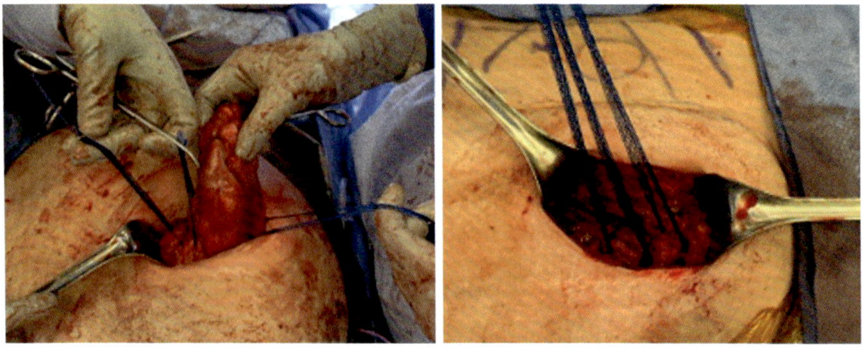

Fig. 11.1 Primary parastomal hernia repair using mesh suture in a figure-of-eight fashion

not routinely performed, a drain can be left in the subcutaneous space if a significant amount of dead space is present.

11.3.4 Mesh-Based Repairs

Mesh-based repairs are preferred to suture repairs when feasible due to improved short- and long-term recurrence outcomes associated with mesh repairs (7.8–34.6% vs. 57.6–69.4% at two-year follow-up) [12, 13]. Overall quality of evidence evaluating postoperative outcomes and complications between techniques remains poor [13], without clear data to support the superiority of a single technique. In general, sublay repairs are considered the most durable option compared to underlay and overlay repairs. However, the choice to use one repair technique over another is nuanced, with consideration given to a variety of technical and clinical factors for each individual patient. The technical aspects of multiple mesh-based repairs, as well as considerations for each technique are described below.

11.3.4.1 Open Onlay Repairs

Open onlay repairs involve placing a piece of mesh over the anterior fascia. This can be performed through a local peristomal incision similar to a primary repair, or by taking down the mucocutaneous junction. Dissection is again carried down to the anterior fascia and the stoma is freed from the surrounding tissue and hernia sac. After reduction of the hernia contents and a resection of the hernia sac, a subcutaneous pocket can be created circumferentially around the stoma, at least 5 cm in all directions. Care should be taken during medial dissection if a separate midline hernia is present to avoid damage to the hernia contents.

The fascial defect should be closed with monofilament or mesh-suture. The mesh is then placed over top following fascial closure using fibrin sealant staples or other fixation techniques. If the stoma required local revision and takedown at the mucocutaneous junction, a cruciate incision can be made to deliver the bowel through the mesh. Additionally, a keyhole configuration can be used if the stoma is left *in situ* (Fig. 11.2). Care should be taken regardless of configuration to ensure the mesh is configurated correctly in relation to the bowel and that the mesh defect does not constrict the bowel or adjacent mesentery. Additionally, the creation of a large subcutaneous pocket to accommodate mesh placement can lead to seroma formation or surgical site infections. A closed suction drain should be left within the subcutaneous space.

11.3.4.2 Minimally Invasive Underlay Repairs

Minimally invasive underlay repairs involve placing an intraperitoneal mesh using a laparoscopic or robotic platform (Fig. 11.3). They have the advantage of allowing for placement of an intraperitoneal piece of mesh, while improving recovery time and wound related morbidity compared to an open overlay repair. The traditional laparoscopic underlay repair involves using transfascial sutures to affix the mesh to the peritoneum and allow for appropriate positioning. A keyhole mesh configuration

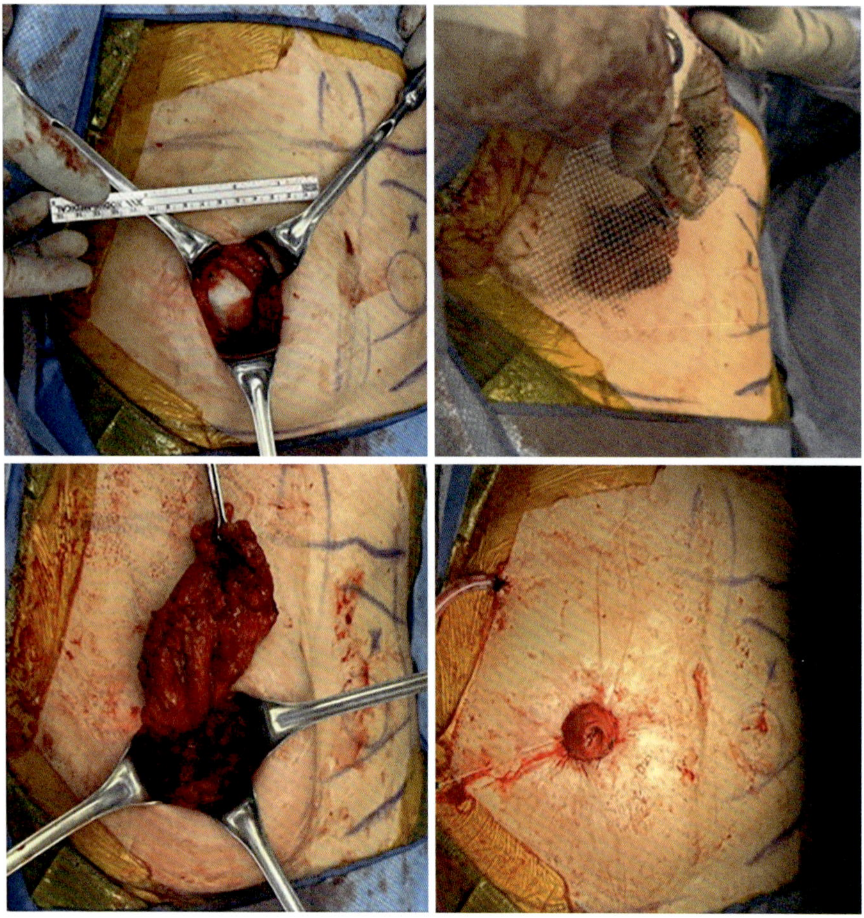

Fig. 11.2 Open onlay mesh repair demonstrating *(top left)* the anterior fascial defect; *(top right)* making of cruciate incision to allow for passage of the revised stoma bowel through mesh; *(bottom left)* cruciate mesh positioned in onlay position over closed anterior fascia (not pictured); *(bottom right)* final maturation of stoma with drain in the subcutaneous space

was traditionally used to place the mesh around the stoma. Repair strength with this technique is limited, however, by the defect created within the mesh and its tendency to enlarge over time as well as the lack of central overlap with the mesh at the defect site. A minimally invasive modified Sugarbaker repair, by contrast, involves placing a flat piece of intraperitoneal mesh in the underlay position. This creates a tunnel of mesh around the stoma bowel and lateralizes the bowel against the abdominal wall.

Whether performing a laparoscopic or robotic repair, the patient should be placed in a supine position with the arms tucked. Abdominal entry can be obtained based upon surgeon preference. We prefer gasless optical entry in the upper quadrant remote from the stoma site. Additional ports can then be placed laterally,

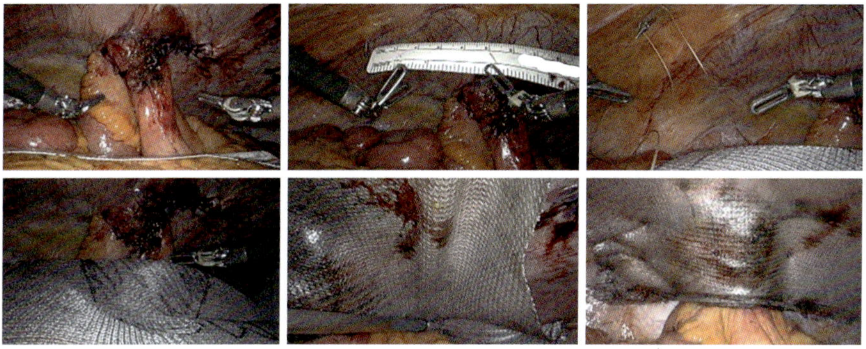

Fig. 11.3 Robotic intraperitoneal underlay (IPUM) Sugarbaker mesh repair demonstrating *(top left)* closure of the fascial defect around the stoma; *(top middle)* measuring placement of cardinal transfascial sutures to ensure appropriate mesh overlap; *(top right)* passage of a transfascial suture to affix the mesh to the anterior abdominal wall; *(bottom left)* mesh configuration after placement of all transfascial sutures; *(bottom middle)* lateralization of the stoma bowel using a laparoscopic tacking device; *(bottom right)* final mesh configuration after complete mesh fixation with tacks

contralateral to the stoma site. Adhesiolysis is performed with judicious energy use, taking care to adequately clear the midline abdominal wall to evaluate for any concomitant midline defects. Once mobilized from surrounding adhesions and nearby bowel, the hernia contents are reduced, and the stoma is further mobilized from the hernia sac. The fascial defect is then measured and closed using a suture passer or suturing the defect closed. The maneuverability gained by the robotic platform allows for defect closure at locations that would be challenging laparoscopically.

If performing an underlay modified Sugarbaker repair, an appropriately sized mesh is placed into the abdominal cavity. A standard technique for mesh positioning involves placing transfascial cardinal sutures through the abdominal wall and mesh, including on either side of the stoma bowel where it enters the mesh. This aids in creating the mesh tunnel for the lateralized bowel to travel through and ensures that additional bowel does slip under the mesh. A tacking device can then secure the mesh to the abdominal wall circumferentially. Care should be taken to ensure the transfascial sutures do not cause strangulation of the stoma bowel and that the bowel is not inadvertently fixated to the abdominal wall with suture or tacks.

For robotic repairs, the stoma bowel may be affixed to the abdominal wall to ensure adequate lateralization and mesh positioning. The mesh can be positioned and fixated to the abdominal wall and lateralized stoma bowel with absorbable barbed suture.

11.3.4.3 Retromuscular Sublay Repairs

Retromuscular sublay repairs are a durable repair option for parastomal hernias that involve placing a piece of mesh in the retromuscular space by performing a posterior component separation with or without an associated transversus abdominis release (TAR). They are a particularly good option for patients who have failed other mesh-based repairs and for patients with a concomitant midline hernia as it allows for a wide mesh overlap of all defects. Configuration of mesh can again be placed in a keyhole or modified Sugarbaker configuration. These repairs are often performed in an open fashion due to the complexity of the hernia defect and repair but can be performed in a minimally invasive fashion.

11.3.4.4 Open Pauli Parastomal Hernia Repair

The Pauli parastomal hernia repair (PPHR) is a retromuscular sublay repair that involves performing a TAR (either ipsilateral to the stoma site or bilaterally) and placing the mesh in a modified Sugarbaker configuration (Fig. 11.4). A midline laparotomy incision is made to gain access into the abdominal cavity and adhesiolysis is performed to free the bowel and omentum from the abdominal wall. The hernia contents are then reduced and the bowel is dissected from the hernia sac and is completely mobilized from all surrounding adhesions. The stoma is left *in situ* without takedown of the mucocutaneous junction. Any previously placed mesh from prior repairs should be excised as able.

The posterior rectus sheath is then incised to enter the retrorectus space. This is then carried out laterally to dissect the posterior sheath away from the rectus, including circumferentially around the stoma site. Care should be taken to identify and protect the neurovascular bundles as the dissection is carried out laterally.

Due to the need for mesh overlap lateral to the stoma, an ipsilateral TAR is then performed. The posterior lamella of the internal oblique and the insertion of the transversus abdominis on the posterior sheath to allow for entry into the pretransversalis space. Inferiorly, this becomes the preperitoneal space below the arcuate line. This incision should be made medial to the linea semilunaris to avoid injury to the neurovascular bundles. Upon entering the pretransversalis plane, this dissection can be carried behind the stoma laterally, superiorly to the costal margin and inferiorly to the space of Retzius. If there is adequate mesh overlap and the midline fascia

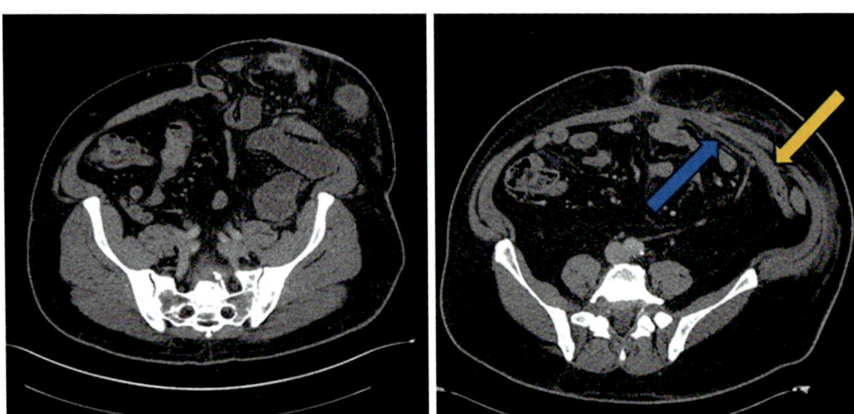

Fig. 11.4 *(left)* Preoperative CT scan of parastomal hernia. *(right)* Postoperative CT scan following Pauli parastomal hernia repair (PPHR) demonstrating lateralized stoma bowel *(yellow arrow)* within the retromuscular space *(blue arrow)*

can be closed without tension, a unilateral TAR is sufficient. However, in cases with a large concomitant midline defect or those where additional mobilization is needed, a contralateral TAR should be performed to ensure appropriate mesh overlap.

After the retromuscular pocket is created, the posterior sheath is incised (lateral, inferolateral or superolateral) to allow for stoma lateralization. Care should be taken to ensure this follows the course of the mesentery to allow for adequate lateralization and avoid ischemia related to twisting of the mesentery. Following lateralization of the stoma, the incision made in the posterior sheath around the stoma as well as the midline posterior sheath is closed.

Mesh is then brought into the retromuscular pocket and oriented in a Sugarbaker configuration with a goal of 8 cm of mesh overlap circumferentially. The mesh can then be secured using suture or fibrin sealant. We recommend leaving a drain within the retromuscular space. The anterior fascia is then closed with absorbable suture. Following skin closure, a closed incisional vacuum dressing can be placed over the incision.

Recurrences following PPHR are often related to lack of adequate lateralization of the stoma bowel. This can be particularly challenging in cases with a short mesentery or in association with ileal conduit hernias, where lateralization may be limited by ureter length. If there is concern for inadequate bowel lateralization intraoperatively, the operative plan should shift to use another mesh configuration.

11.3.4.5 Open Keyhole/Cruciate Repair

A keyhole mesh configuration can be performed in scenarios where the surgeon does not feel that the bowel can be adequately lateralized to achieve a retromuscular Sugarbaker repair. Additionally, if the stoma needs to be taken down at the mucocutaneous junction to be revised or relocated to a new site, a cruciate configuration can be used as this is less technically challenging. The retromuscular dissection with TAR is undertaken in a similar manner to the open PPHR. No bowel lateralization within the posterior sheath is needed and the mesh can be configured around the bowel in a keyhole (if left *in situ*) or cruciate (if revised) fashion.

Long-term outcomes comparing sublay mesh configurations are limited. One study found the recurrence rate following PPHR was 10.7% compared to 30.4% for keyhole/cruciate configurations but was underpowered to detect a statistically significant difference based on configuration [14]. Additionally, a recent randomized clinical trial sought to evaluate recurrence rates between retromuscular mesh configurations. This study found that Sugarbaker mesh placement was non-superior to keyhole repairs [15]. However, criticism regarding selection bias and randomization of patients as well as differences in the rates of follow-up between the groups. Further long-term regarding these repairs study is needed.

11.3.4.6 Minimally Invasive Retromuscular Repair

While first described in an open manner, the PPHR repair can be performed using minimally invasive techniques in surgeons with appropriate expertise. Minimally invasive approaches follow the same general techniques as an open PPHR: dissection of the retrorectus space and TAR by incising medial to the semilunar line to

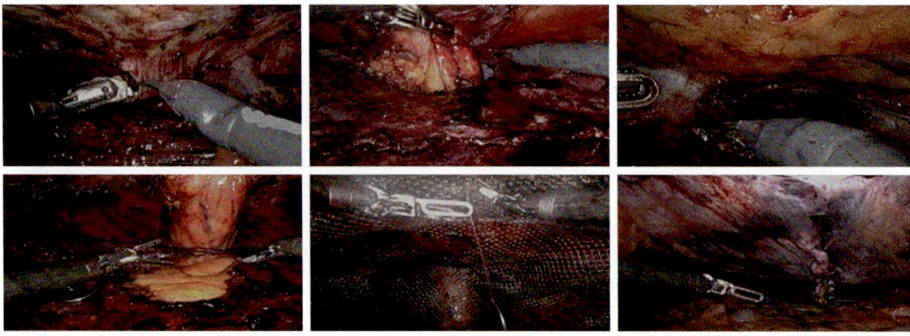

Fig. 11.5 *(top left)* Incision of the medial insertion of the posterior rectus sheath. *(top middle)* Location of the stoma at the lateral border of the rectus with need for additional mesh coverage. *(top right)* Incision of the posterior lamella of the internal oblique to start the ipsilateral transversus abdominis release (TAR). *(bottom left)* Lateralized stoma bowel within the retromuscular space with closure of the posterior sheath. *(bottom middle)* Retromuscular placement of mesh in a Sugarbaker configuration. *(bottom right)* Intra-abdominal view of the completed repair following flap closure

preserve the neurovascular bundles, lateralization of the stoma bowel by incising the posterior sheath in the direction of the bowl mesentery, and placement of a retrorectus mesh in a Sugarbaker (or keyhole) configuration (Fig. 11.5).

Two approaches can be used to enter the retrorectus space: a transabdominal approach and an extended-view totally extraperitoneal (eTEP) repair, which allows direct entry into the preperitoneal plane without abdominal entry. This is usually performed via optical entry directly into the retrorectus space contralateral to the stoma site. For both a transabdominal and eTEP approach, additional working ports are placed laterally on the contralateral side from the stoma. If a bilateral TAR is needed to facilitate mesh overlap or fascial closure in the presence of a large midline defect, the robot will need to be undocked and ports placed on the opposite side.

11.4 Conclusion

Parastomal hernias are common following stoma creation. Multiple technical and clinical considerations must be undertaken when selecting the optimal repair type. Long-term data evaluating the optimal repair technique is needed.

References

1. Carne PWG, Robertson GM, Frizelle FA. Parastomal hernia. Br J Surg. 2003;90(7):784–93.
2. Correa Marinez A, Bock D, Erestam S, et al. Methods of colostomy construction: no effect on parastomal hernia rate. Results from stoma-const – a randomized controlled trial. Ann Surg. 2021;273(4):640–7.
3. Gavigan T, Rozario N, Matthews B, Reinke C. Trends in parastomal hernia repair in the United States: a 14-y review. J Surg Res. 2017;218:78–85.

4. Malik TAM, Lee MJ, Harikrishnan AB. The incidence of stoma related morbidity – a systematic review of randomised controlled trials. Ann R Coll Surg Engl. 2018;100(7):501–8.
5. Krishnamurty DM, Blatnik J, Mutch M. Stoma complications. Clin Colon Rectal Surg. 2017;30(3):193–200.
6. Antoniou SA, Agresta F, Garcia Alamino JM, et al. European Hernia Society guidelines on prevention and treatment of parastomal hernias. Hernia. 2018;22(1):183–98.
7. Davis BR, Valente MA, Goldberg JE, et al. The American Society of Colon and Rectal Surgeons clinical practice guidelines for ostomy surgery. Dis Colon Rectum. 2022;65(10):1173–90.
8. Kroese LF, Lambrichts DPV, Jeekel J, et al. Non-operative treatment as a strategy for patients with parastomal hernia: a multicentre, retrospective cohort study. Color Dis. 2018;20(6):545–51.
9. Howard R, Rob F, Thumma J, et al. Contemporary outcomes of elective parastomal hernia repair in older adults. JAMA Surg. 2023;158(4):394–402.
10. Fleming AM, Phillips AL, Drake JA, et al. Sugarbaker versus keyhole repair for parastomal hernia: a systematic review and meta-analysis of comparative studies. J Gastrointest Surg. 2023;27(3):573–84.
11. Quattrone M, Moyer ED, Zolin SJ, et al. Short-term outcomes of mesh-suture repair in the treatment of ventral hernias: a single-center study. Surg Endosc. 2025;39(3):2129–35.
12. Al Shakarchi J, Williams JG. Systematic review of open techniques for parastomal hernia repair. Tech Coloproctol. 2014;18(5):427–32.
13. Hansson BME, Slater NJ, van der Velden AS, et al. Surgical techniques for parastomal hernia repair: a systematic review of the literature. Ann Surg. 2012;255(4):685–95.
14. Miller BT, Krpata DM, Petro CC, et al. Biologic vs synthetic mesh for parastomal hernia repair: post hoc analysis of a multicenter randomized controlled trial. J Am Coll Surg. 2022;235(3):401–9.
15. Maskal SM, Ellis RC, Fafaj A, et al. Open retromuscular Sugarbaker vs keyhole mesh placement for parastomal hernia repair. JAMA Surg. 2024;159(9):982–9.

Part III

Special Scenarios and Challenges

Management of Enterocutaneous and Abdominal Fistulas

12

Carlo Sagnelli

12.1 Enterocutaneous Fistulas: Introduction

Enterocutaneous fistulas (ECFs) present a significant challenge in abdominal wall surgery, often complicating postoperative recovery and requiring meticulous management. These fistulas are abnormal connections between the gastrointestinal (GI) tract and the skin, leading to fluid loss, infection risk, and impaired wound healing. Their successful management involves a multidisciplinary approach, including optimization of the patient's nutritional status, infection control, fluid and electrolyte balance, wound care, and, when necessary, surgical intervention [1, 2].

12.2 Etiology and Risk Factors

ECFs commonly arise as complications of abdominal surgery, particularly in patients with [2]:

- Postoperative complications (anastomotic leaks, intra-abdominal infections)
- Previous abdominal surgeries leading to adhesions and compromised intestinal integrity
- Malignancies involving the GI tract
- Inflammatory bowel disease such as Crohn's disease
- Radiation enteritis causing tissue ischemia and fibrosis
- Abdominal trauma or spontaneous fistula formation due to sepsis or ischemia.

C. Sagnelli (✉)
Department of General Surgery, A.O.R.N. dei Colli Monaldi Hospital, Naples, Italy
e-mail: carlo.sagnelli@ospedalideicolli.it

D. Cuccurullo, C. Rispoli (eds.), *Complex Abdominal Wall Surgery*, Updates in Surgery, https://doi.org/10.1007/978-3-032-24284-6_12

12.2.1 Classification of Enterocutaneous Fistulas

ECFs are classified based on their output and anatomical location [2]:

- By output:
  - Low-output fistulas (<200 mL/day): typically easier to manage non-surgically
  - Moderate-output fistulas (200–500 mL/day): require careful fluid and nutritional management
  - High-output fistulas (>500 mL/day): associated with significant metabolic disturbances and high morbidity.
- By anatomical location:
  - Proximal (stomach, duodenum, jejunum): associated with high fluid loss
  - Distal (ileum, colon): often have lower output and may allow for spontaneous closure.

12.2.2 Initial Management and Stabilization

The initial phase of management focuses on sepsis control, fluid resuscitation, and nutritional support [2, 3].

- Sepsis control: broad-spectrum antibiotics should be initiated based on suspected bacterial flora and de-escalated once cultures are available.
- Source control is crucial. Percutaneous drainage of abscesses or infected collections can prevent systemic complications.
- Fluid and electrolyte management: high-output fistulas result in significant fluid, sodium, potassium, and bicarbonate losses, requiring aggressive replacement. Regular monitoring of serum electrolytes, renal function, and acid-base balance is necessary.
- Nutritional optimization: total parenteral nutrition (TPN) is preferred in high-output ECFs to minimize GI secretions and promote healing. In select cases, enteral feeding distal to the fistula may be possible and beneficial. Correction of malnutrition (albumin, prealbumin levels) improves surgical outcomes.

12.2.3 Wound and Fistula Management

- Skin protection and local care: the presence of corrosive enteric effluent requires effective stoma appliances, wound barriers, and negative pressure wound therapy (NPWT) or vacuum-assisted closure (VAC) therapy, to prevent skin breakdown. Frequent assessment of periwound skin is crucial to prevent complications such as maceration and secondary infection.

- NPWT or VAC therapy: NPWT, also known as VAC therapy, has become an essential tool in the management of complex ECFs, especially when associated with open abdomen or significant abdominal wall defects. The primary goals are control of fistula effluent, protection of the surrounding skin, promotion of granulation tissue formation, and optimization of conditions for eventual surgical repair [3, 4].
- Mechanism of action: NPWT applies continuous or intermittent sub-atmospheric pressure to the wound through a sealed dressing connected to a vacuum system. This:
  - Reduces fistula output by lowering intra-abdominal pressure and isolating the fistula.
  - Promotes angiogenesis and granulation tissue formation.
  - Decreases local edema and bacterial colonization.
  - Protects the periwound skin from corrosive enteric effluents [5].

In high-output fistulas, standard NPWT may be challenging. Advanced techniques and devices may improve outcomes: custom-designed ostomy rings, pouches, or silicone adapters integrated into the NPWT dressing divert effluent away from the wound bed; fistula output is collected separately, preventing maceration and maintaining dressing efficacy; use of hydrocolloid barriers or stoma appliances enhances seal integrity [6].

12.2.4 Clinical Outcomes and Benefits of VAC-Assisted NPWT

Recent studies demonstrate significant clinical benefits associated with VAC-assisted NPWT in patients with abdominal wall defects and fistulas:

- Improved infection control: NPWT facilitates continuous removal of contaminated exudate, decreasing bacterial colonization and enhancing local sepsis control.
- Reduction in morbidity and mortality: when applied as a bridge to definitive surgery, NPWT has been shown to decrease morbidity and improve survival rates, particularly in critically ill patients.
- Enhanced patient comfort and reduced nursing workload: by decreasing the frequency of dressing changes, VAC systems improve patient tolerance and simplify nursing care.
- Promotion of spontaneous fistula closure: in low- to moderate-output fistulas (<500 mL/day), NPWT may enhance spontaneous closure rates by optimizing granulation tissue formation and maintaining a controlled wound environment [4, 5].

12.2.5 Limitations and Considerations

Despite its numerous benefits, NPWT requires careful application and patient selection:

- Avoidance of direct bowel contact: NPWT should never be applied directly over exposed bowel loops without protective interfaces, such as non-adherent dressings or specially designed fistula isolation systems.
- Management of high-output fistulas: in cases of high-output fistulas (>500 mL/day), NPWT alone may be insufficient. Combined therapy with parenteral nutrition, octreotide, or somatostatin analogues is often required to reduce effluent and promote healing. Continuous monitoring of fluid balance, electrolytes, and nutritional status is essential to avoid metabolic derangements and ensure optimal recovery [7].
- Layered dressing techniques: combining foam dressings with non-adherent interfaces and protective stomas can prevent fistula enlargement and facilitate control of output [6, 7].

12.2.6 Future Perspectives

Emerging evidence suggests that integrating NPWT with advanced biomaterials, tissue-engineered scaffolds, and regenerative therapies could further improve outcomes in patients with complex fistulas and large abdominal wall defects. Ongoing clinical trials are investigating the synergistic effects of NPWT with stem cell therapy and negative pressure instillation systems.

Ultimately, it can be concluded that the best results are achieved when combininig:

- Aggressive sepsis control
- Nutritional optimization (preferably TPN) with high caloric intake
- NPWT to manage fluid output
- Delayed surgical reconstruction when spontaneous closure fails.

12.2.7 Definitive Surgical Management

Once the patient is stabilized, elective surgical repair is considered if the fistula does not close spontaneously within 6–12 weeks [7]. The surgical approach depends on:

- Location and anatomy of the fistula
- Presence of adhesions, inflammation, or abscesses
- Status of the abdominal wall (previous mesh repair, hernias, or loss of domain).

12.2.8 Key Surgical Principles

- Fistula resection with bowel reanastomosis preferred if healthy bowel margins are present.
- Segmental resection for diseased bowel in Crohn's disease or radiation enteritis.

- Abdominal wall reconstruction using biologic, biosynthetic, or hybrid meshes with component separation techniques when needed [2, 7, 8].

12.2.9 Postoperative Care and Long-Term Considerations

Early enteral feeding should be attempted to enhance gut recovery. Ongoing nutritional support and rehabilitation are essential to prevent recurrence. Long-term follow-up is required to monitor for recurrent fistulas, stricture formation and incisional hernias.

12.2.10 Conclusions

Management of ECFs in abdominal wall surgery requires a systematic, multidisciplinary approach. Early recognition, aggressive stabilization, optimal wound care, and carefully planned surgical intervention are essential to reduce morbidity and improve outcomes.

Advances in nutritional therapy, NPWT techniques, and the use of biosynthetic or hybrid meshes in reconstructive surgery have significantly enhanced prognosis for these complex patients [9, 10].

12.3 Enteroatmospheric Fistulas: Introduction

Enteroatmospheric fistulas (EAFs) are one of the most formidable complications encountered in open abdomen scenarios, characterized by direct communication between the GI tract and the external environment through an unclosed abdominal wound. They carry high morbidity and mortality, and their management mandates a multidisciplinary, evidence-informed, stepwise approach.

12.3.1 Definition

EAF is defined as a pathological opening in the intestinal lumen that communicates directly with the atmosphere. It is characterized by the absence of a defined fistula tract and a lack of well-vascularized surrounding tissue, which significantly impairs spontaneous healing. EAFs most commonly occur within an open abdomen, usually following abdominal trauma, sepsis, or complications of laparotomy, where the protective barriers of the abdominal wall are disrupted. EAFs are associated with the direct spillage of enteric contents into the open peritoneal cavity, leading to a high risk of contamination, infection, and severe complications. The surrounding tissue is typically poorly vascularized, which significantly compromises spontaneous closure and makes surgical management challenging (Fig. 12.1).

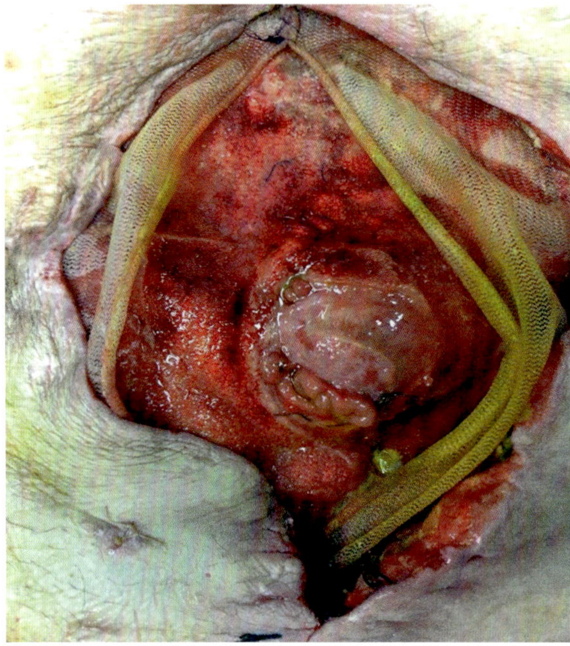

Fig. 12.1 Enteroatmospheric fistula in the presence of a biosynthetic mesh

One of the hallmark features is the free spillage of enteric contents into the open peritoneal cavity, predisposing patients to peritoneal contamination, persistent infection, and severe fluid-electrolyte imbalances. Because of these anatomical and pathophysiological characteristics, EAFs represent one of the most complex and life-threatening complications in abdominal wall and gastrointestinal surgery.

According to the World Society of Emergency Surgery (WSES) guideline, preventive strategies are essential. These include early fascial closure, protection of exposed bowel with coverings (plastic sheets, omentum, skin), avoidance of synthetic mesh or NPWT directly on viscera, and deep burying of intestinal anastomoses to reduce EAF risk (Grade 1C of the abovementioned guidelines) [7, 9].

12.3.2 Classification of Enteroatmospheric Fistulas

- Based on output:
  - Low: <200 mL/day
  - Moderate: 200–500 mL/day
  - High: >500 mL/day.
- According to the Björck classification (adapted by WSACS): considers adhesions and open abdomen context, but more complex composite schemes also exist that factor in location, number, exposure, and output [9].

12.3.3 Initial Management: Resuscitation, Nutrition, and Infection Control

- Resuscitation: address fluid/electrolyte imbalances and nitrogen/protein losses, which are substantial in open abdomen and EAF scenarios (estimated 2 g N per liter of fluid lost).
- Nutritional support: initiate TPN immediately post-resuscitation (Grade 1C—WSES guideline). Early enteral nutrition is preferred if feasible and distal feeding is accessibile but high-output fistulas may preclude its use (Grade 2C—WSES guideline).
- Sepsis control: antibiotics therapy and drainage or source control are mandatory [2, 7].

12.3.4 Effluent Isolation and Wound Management

Effective isolation of fistula effluent is critical for promoting granulation and protecting surrounding skin [4, 6, 7].

NPWT, in its various configurations, is the most widely accepted modality to manage EAF within an open abdomen: it facilitates wound healing, granulation, and conversion to controlled enterostomy; definitive repair should follow complete recovery (typically after ≥6 months) [5, 7, 10].

As stated above in the ECF section, various custom-designed sistems (Fistula Solution®, floating stoma, etc.) exist to divert effluent away from the wound bed and promote healing through VAC.

Recent innovations include fistula patches, fistuloclysis, 3D-printed stents, injection-molded stents, and covered stents, each offering anatomical customization and improved isolation, but still largely experimental with limited clinical validation [6, 10] (Fig. 12.2).

12.3.5 Temporary Abdominal Closure and Timing of Definitive Repair

Leading guidelines (WSES, Abdominal Compartment Society [WSACS], Eastern Association for the Surgery of Trauma [EAST], National Institute for Health and Care Excellence [NICE]) endorse NPWT as the preferred temporary abdominal closure (TAC) approach to optimize fascial closure, reduce abdominal compartment syndrome, and minimize fistula formation. Aim for definitive fascial closure within 7–10 days, when clinically possible [5, 7, 11].

The European Hernia Society (EHS) advises dynamic closure techniques (e.g., mesh-mediated fascial traction, dynamic sutures) over static methods; however, these must be individualized and cautious in contaminated fields due to infection risk.

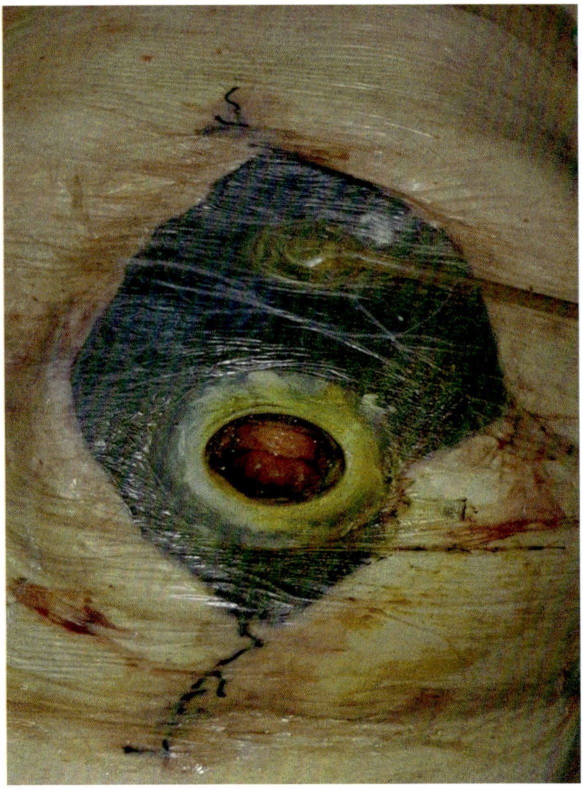

Fig. 12.2 Negative pressure wound therapy (NPWT) with a fistula management solution in an enteroatmospheric fistula

Ultimately, definitive interventions, fistula resection, restoration of intestinal continuity, and abdominal wall reconstruction, should be delayed until patient recovery and wound maturation, often at least 6 months post-event.

12.3.6 Surgical Options and Limitations in the Management of EAFs

In selected patients with EAFs or complex abdominal wall defects, it may be considered to perform a bowel resection to remove the affected segment or to create a proximal bowel diversion in order to control contamination and reduce the risk of ongoing sepsis.

However, these approaches are often not feasible in the acute setting due to several anatomical and physiological constraints:

- Mesenteric retraction and edema: severe inflammation and mesenteric shortening make bowel mobilization technically challenging and increase the risk of vascular injury.

- Frozen abdomen: extensive adhesions and dense fibrotic tissue prevent safe dissection and manipulation of intestinal loops.
- Loss of abdominal domain: retraction of the abdominal wall and visceral edema may significantly reduce the available intra-abdominal space, complicating primary closure and increasing the risk of abdominal compartment syndrome.

Because of these limitations, delayed surgical strategies combined with optimized supportive care are often preferred until local and systemic conditions are stabilized.

One of the primary goals of therapy should be to convert an EAF into an ECF, with the ultimate aim of planning a delayed surgical reconstruction (Fig. 12.3).

At the time of surgical reconstruction, we should be able to resect the fistulous segment, restore bowel continuity, and reconstruct the abdominal wall (e.g., component separation, use of meshes).

Preoperative optimization of modifiable risk factors—nutrition, infections, lifestyle—is crucial to reduce recurrence [2, 7].

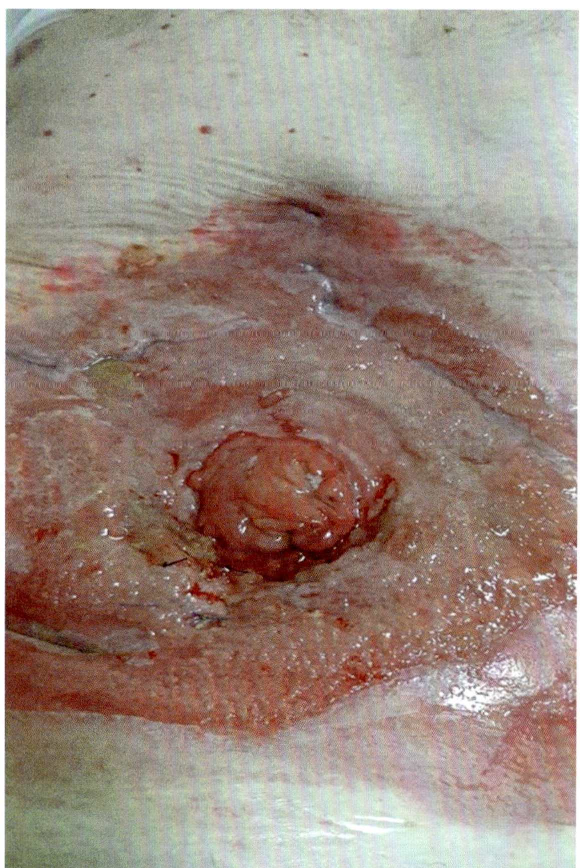

Fig. 12.3 Conversion of an enteroatmospheric fistula into an enterocutaneous fistula

12.3.7 Conclusions

Management of EAF in the setting of abdominal wall surgery demands a systematic, phased, and guideline-informed strategy. Best practices emphasize:

- Rigorous prevention and protection measures
- Early and appropriate nutritional and sepsis control
- Efficient wound and effluent management, primarily via NPWT
- Timely, but safe, fascial closure, supported by dynamic techniques when possible
- Delayed, definitive surgical repair in a non-inflamed, optimized patient.

This structured, evidence-based approach, supported by WSES, WSACS, EHS, and current literature, provides a robust framework to improve outcomes in this challenging field [1, 5, 9–11].

12.4 Use of Biosynthetic and Hybrid Meshes in Abdominal Wall Reconstruction for ECFs and EAFs

Biosynthetic and hybrid meshes have emerged as valuable tools in abdominal wall reconstruction, particularly in the challenging context of ECF and EAF, where surgical fields are frequently contaminated or potentially infected. Unlike permanent synthetic prostheses, biosynthetic meshes are designed to provide temporary reinforcement, gradually resorbing as native tissue regenerates, thereby reducing the long-term infectious burden and facilitating collagen deposition and neovascularization. These properties make them suitable for complex abdominal wall repairs, especially when biologic meshes are unavailable or cost-prohibitive [8, 12–14].

Biosynthetic meshes have been developed to combine the advantages of synthetic and biologic prostheses, offering both mechanical strength and enhanced biocompatibility. They can be manufactured from different materials, including monofilament macroporous poly-4-hydroxybutyrate (e.g., Phasix®), three-dimensional scaffolds composed of polyglycolic acid and trimethylene carbonate (e.g., Bio-A®), or multifilament meshes derived from trimethylene carbonate and polylactic acid (e.g., TIGR® Matrix). These prostheses provide handling characteristics, fixation, and tensile strength comparable to permanent synthetic meshes, while undergoing complete hydrolysis within 6–18 months depending on the specific material, leaving no residual foreign body. Their high biocompatibility ensures minimal foreign body reaction and, together with their ability to promote bacterial clearance, results in a reduced risk of infection. Despite these benefits, potential drawbacks have been reported, such as the development of seromas or hematomas, and a risk of hernia recurrence when resorption occurs too rapidly. Moreover, due to their resorbable nature, biosynthetic meshes are not recommended for implantation in already infected fields, where biologic prostheses may represent a more reliable option.

Hybrid meshes, on the other hand, combine the structural durability of permanent macroporous scaffolds with biologic or resorbable components that enhance tissue integration and decrease susceptibility to chronic infection. Two principal designs are currently used:

- Hybrid composite meshes (e.g., GORE® SYNECOR), integrating a permanent synthetic scaffold with bioresorbable layers or anti-adhesion coatings, enabling intraperitoneal or preperitoneal placement while minimizing adhesion formation and infection risk [12, 15].
- Reinforced biologic meshes (e.g., OviTex®), consisting of an extracellular biologic matrix reinforced with polymer filaments, intended to balance mechanical strength with improved biologic incorporation and reduced infectious complications [16].

Successful integration of these prosthetic devices requires a staged surgical approach. During the acute phase, as has been extensively discussed in the preceding paragraphs, the therapeutic focus should be on sepsis control, effluent isolation, often achieved using NPWT with dedicated fistula-isolation techniques, nutritional optimization, and stabilization of electrolyte and metabolic balance. Definitive abdominal wall reconstruction should be delayed until local inflammation has resolved, tissue planes are adequately vascularized, and systemic conditions are optimized. At the time of surgical reconstruction, retrorectus (sublay) mesh placement is generally preferred, as it maximizes tissue integration and minimizes the risk of infection and fistula recurrence. Bridging techniques, where fascial approximation is not possible, should be reserved for selected cases and approached cautiously, as they are associated with higher recurrence rates [2, 8, 12–15, 17].

Clinical evidence suggests that both biosynthetic and hybrid meshes demonstrate lower rates of chronic infection and mesh explantation compared with permanent synthetics, while maintaining comparable recurrence profiles to biologic meshes but at a significantly lower cost. Furthermore, reinforced biologic meshes and hybrid composites have shown favorable outcomes in contaminated and complex fields, including scenarios involving ECF and EAF, where prosthetic salvage is often possible even in the presence of localized infection when managed conservatively with drainage, antibiotics, and NPWT.

Nevertheless, several limitations remain. These devices are not completely immune to infection, and their long-term durability is inferior to that of permanent synthetics, making careful patient selection essential. Optimal results depend on achieving sepsis control, ensuring adequate nutrition, and selecting the appropriate device and placement strategy based on defect size, contamination grade, and visceral exposure risk. Whenever intraperitoneal placement is necessary, the use of barrier-coated hybrid meshes in conjunction with visceral separation techniques is strongly recommended.

In summary, biosynthetic and hybrid meshes represent an effective and versatile option for abdominal wall reconstruction in patients with ECF and EAF once contamination has been controlled and local tissue conditions optimized. Their integration within a multimodal strategy, including NPWT, staged reconstruction, and multidisciplinary care, offers the potential for reduced infectious complications, lower recurrence rates, and improved long-term outcomes. However, further high-quality comparative studies are required to define optimal timing, patient selection criteria, and device choice in this complex patient population [12, 14, 15, 17].

References

1. Pepe G, Chiarello MM, Bianchi V, et al. Entero-cutaneous and entero-atmospheric fistulas: insights into management using negative pressure wound therapy. J Clin Med. 2024;13(5):1279.
2. Schecter WP. Management of enterocutaneous fistulas. Surg Clin North Am. 2011;91(3):481–91.
3. Demetriades D, Salim A. Management of the open abdomen. Surg Clin North Am. 2014;94(1):131–53.
4. Terzi C, Egeli T, Canda AE, Arslan NC. Management of enteroatmospheric fistulae. Int Wound J. 2014;11 Suppl 1((Suppl 1)):17–21.
5. Coccolini F, Sartelli M, Sawyer R, et al. Source control in emergency general surgery: WSES, GAIS, SIS-E, SIS – a guidelines. World J Emerg Surg. 2023;18(1):41.
6. Huang J, Ren H, Jiang Y, et al. Technique advances in enteroatmospheric fistula isolation after open abdomen: a review and outlook. Front Surg. 2021;7:559443.
7. Coccolini F, Roberts D, Ansaloni L, et al. The open abdomen in trauma and non-trauma patients: WSES guidelines. World J Emerg Surg. 2018;13:7.
8. Piccoli M, Agresta F, Attinà GM, et al. "Complex abdominal wall" management: evidence-based guidelines of the Italian consensus conference. Updat Surg. 2019;71(2):255–72.
9. Seternes A, Rekstad LC, Mo S, et al. Open abdomen treated with negative pressure wound therapy: indications, management and survival. World J Surg. 2017;41(1):152–61.
10. Bobkiewicz A, Walczak D, Smoliński S, et al. Management of enteroatmospheric fistula with negative pressure wound therapy in open abdomen treatment: a multicentre observational study. Int Wound J. 2017;14(1):255–64.
11. Diaz JJ Jr, Dutton WD, Ott MM, et al. Eastern Association for the Surgery of Trauma: a review of the management of the open abdomen – part 2 "Management of the open abdomen". J Trauma. 2011;71(2):502–12.
12. Goetz M, Jurczyk M, Junger H, et al. Semiresorbable biologic hybrid meshes for ventral abdominal hernia repair in potentially contaminated settings: lower risk of recurrence. Updat Surg. 2022;74(6):1995–2001.
13. Sivaraj D, Fischer KS, Kim TS, et al. Outcomes of biosynthetic and synthetic mesh in ventral hernia repair. Plast Reconstr Surg Glob Open. 2022;10(12):e4707.
14. Carbonell AM, Criss CN, Cobb WS, et al. Outcomes of synthetic mesh in contaminated ventral hernia repairs. J Am Coll Surg. 2013;217(6):991–8.
15. Goldblatt MI, Reynolds M, Doerhoff CR, et al. Ventral hernia repair with a hybrid absorbable-permanent preperitoneal mesh. Surg Laparosc Endosc Percutan Tech. 2024;34(6):596–602.
16. Al-Qudimat AR, Altahtamouni SB, Singh K, et al. Clinical outcome of OviTex reinforced tissue matrix in hernia repair: a systematic review and meta-analysis. Qatar Med J. 2025;2025(1):22.
17. Pereira B, Duchesne J, Concon-Filho A, Leppãniemi A. Entero-atmospheric fistula migration: a new management alternative for complex septic open abdomen. Anaesthesiol Intensive Ther. 2020;52(1):56–62.

Abdominal Wall Surgery in Obese and Bariatric Patients: Specific Challenges and Tailored Techniques

13

Rossana Daniela Berta and Galyna Shabat

13.1 Introduction

Obesity has reached epidemic proportions globally and represents one of the most important risk factors for abdominal wall pathology.

The association between obesity and ventral hernia is well established. Large population-based studies demonstrate that obese individuals have a two- to three-fold higher risk of hernia formation and recurrence after repair compared with their non-obese counterparts [1].

Ventral hernias, both primary and incisional, are more frequent in bariatric patients, with prevalence reaching up to 8–10% [2]. The altered biomechanical forces exerted by central adiposity, together with metabolic comorbidities such as diabetes and impaired wound healing, significantly complicate surgical management.

The increasing prevalence of bariatric surgery—with hundreds of thousands of procedures performed annually worldwide—has created a subgroup of patients who often present with both obesity-related comorbidities and abdominal wall defects, either prior to or after weight reduction. Abdominal wall surgery in obese and bariatric patients therefore represents a complex surgical challenge, requiring careful planning, multidisciplinary collaboration, and tailored operative strategies balancing hernia management with weight loss surgery (Fig. 13.1). The goals are to minimize perioperative morbidity, optimize long-term recurrence rates, and integrate abdominal wall reconstruction into the broader framework of weight loss and metabolic improvement.

R. D. Berta (✉)
Bariatric Surgery Unit, IRCCS Policlinico San Donato, Milan, Italy
e-mail: rossanaberta@gmail.com

G. Shabat
Division of General and Foregut Surgery, Department of Biomedical Sciences for Health, IRCCS Policlinico San Donato, University of Milan, Milan, Italy

D. Cuccurullo, C. Rispoli (eds.), *Complex Abdominal Wall Surgery*, Updates in Surgery, https://doi.org/10.1007/978-3-032-24284-6_13

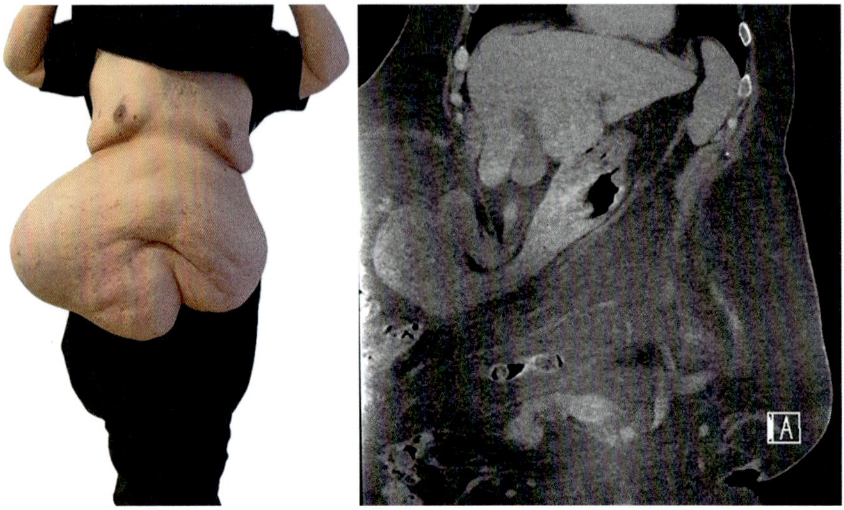

Fig. 13.1 Loss of domain (LOD) in a Class III obese patient with flank hernia

13.2 Background and Clinical Relevance

Obesity (BMI $\geq$30 kg/m^2) is now among the most powerful and prevalent risk factors for primary and incisional herniation. Mechanistically, central adiposity increases intra-abdominal pressure and saps the abdominal wall of functional integrity through altered collagen turnover, chronic low-grade inflammation, and impaired microperfusion. Obesity also clusters with diabetes, obstructive sleep apnea, nonalcoholic fatty liver disease, venous thromboembolism (VTE) risk, and reduced cardiorespiratory reserve—each amplifying perioperative hazard [3, 4].

In parallel, bariatric operations (most commonly sleeve gastrectomy and Roux-en-Y gastric bypass) have risen steeply, improving weight and metabolic disease but introducing new timing questions for hernia repair. Many patients present symptomatic hernias at the time of planned bariatric surgery, while others develop incisional or port-site hernias after massive weight loss. The practicing surgeon therefore requires a framework that integrates hernia biology, timing relative to weight loss, and operative technique.

13.3 Pathophysiology of the Obese Abdominal Wall

Mechanical load and pressure: central obesity elevates baseline intra-abdominal pressure and cough/strain peaks, increasing suture line tension and parietal stress. This favors dehiscence, seroma formation and recurrence [5].

Matrix biology: hyperglycemia, insulin resistance, and systemic inflammation impair fibroblast function, shift collagen I/III ratios toward weaker scar, and reduce crosslinking. This translates clinically into delayed healing and lower tensile strength [6].

Microcirculation and soft tissue envelope. Thick pannus and adipose-rich subcutaneous layers have poorer perfusion and higher dead space, predisposing to surgical site occurrence (SSOs). After massive weight loss, redundant skin and attenuated fascia further complicate closure mechanics.

Nutritional paradox: despite caloric excess, obese patients may have protein-energy malnutrition and micronutrient deficiencies, worsening wound healing [7].

Pulmonary physiology and anesthesia: reduced functional residual capacity, obstructive sleep apnea/obesity hypoventilation syndrome (OSA/OHS), and difficult airways increase perioperative respiratory events and demand tailored anesthesia, positioning and postoperative ventilation strategies.

13.4 Impact of Obesity on Outcomes

Multiple studies confirm that obesity is a predictor of adverse outcomes after ventral hernia repair [4, 5, 8]:

- Higher wound morbidity (surgical site infection, seroma, delayed healing).
- Increased recurrence rates, particularly if BMI remains high at the time of repair.
- Longer operative times and greater resource utilization.

Moszkowicz et al. in a French national registry study demonstrated that patients undergoing hernia repair before bariatric surgery had significantly worse outcomes compared with those who underwent staged or concomitant strategies, emphasizing the importance of timing [1].

13.5 Risk Stratification and Preoperative Optimization

13.5.1 Patient Assessment

- Anthropometrics: BMI is a coarse surrogate; distribution (central vs. peripheral) and waist circumference correlate better with pressure loads.
- Comorbidities: Diabetes (HbA_{1c}), hypertension, OSA (screening with STOP-BANG questionnaire and CPAP adherence), cardiovascular status, smoking, chronic steroid use.
- Nutritional state: Protein status (albumin/prealbumin trends), vitamin D, iron, B12, folate—particularly in post-bariatric patients.
- Hernia phenotype: Defect size and number, loss of domain (LOD), prior mesh, contamination history, fistula/ostomy, skin quality.

13.5.2 Optimization Pillars of Bariatric and Hernia Surgery

- Weight reduction: Even 5–10% loss decreases SSOs and facilitates minimally invasive access; larger reductions (post-bariatric) in hernia repair meaningfully cut recurrence.
- Glycemic control: Target individualized, often HbA_{1c} < 7–8% prior to elective repair; perioperative insulin protocols reduce infectious complications.
- Smoking: Complete cessation ≥4 weeks (longer is better) reduces wound morbidity.
- OSA & pulmonary rehab: Formal OSA evaluation; perioperative CPAP; incentive spirometry and early mobilization.
- Nutrition: Aim for protein 1.2–1.5 g/kg ideal body weight/day; correct micronutrient deficits (vitamin D, iron, B12) common after bariatric operations.
- VTE prevention: Stratify risk; use pharmacologic prophylaxis and early ambulation; consider extended prophylaxis in very high-risk patients.
- Enhanced Recovery After Surgery (ERAS®) pathways: Carbohydrate loading (if not decompensated diabetic), multimodal analgesia, opioid minimization, judicious fluids.

Optimization is not optional: it is part of the operation [8–11].

13.6 GLP-1 Analogues and Ventral Hernia Repair

By significantly reducing excess weight, the use of glucagon-like peptide-1 (GLP-1) analogs could play an important role in the prehabilitation of obese patients undergoing incisional hernia surgery, in whom bariatric surgery is not indicated, in order to reduce postoperative morbidity. There is a growing body of literature, particularly in bariatrics, examining the utility of GLP-1 agonists as a tool for perioperative weight management in surgical patients. GLP-1 treatment should be part of a comprehensive prehabilitation plan that also includes smoking cessation and physiotherapy for respiratory and abdominal muscles.

Preliminary studies indicate their efficacy and safety in facilitating weight loss before incisional hernia repair in patients with severe obesity. While promising, more extensive research is needed to evaluate the safety and efficacy of GLP-1 agonists and long-term impact of these medications on hernia-related outcomes, including hernia recurrence [12, 13].

13.7 Timing of Ventral Hernia Repair Relative to Bariatric Surgery

The presence of a complex ventral hernia in a patient eligible for bariatric surgery presents specific surgical, clinical, and management challenges. A complex ventral hernia is characterized by significant size, recurrences, loss of abdominal domain, multiple adhesions, or involvement of vital structures.

The optimal sequencing of bariatric and hernia surgery remains controversial. Three strategies are currently used:

- Staged strategy/bariatric first, hernia later, preferred in most cases:
  - Rationale: reduce BMI, lower SSOs and recurrence, expand the range of minimally invasive options and convert complex to standard repairs.
  - Indications: large defects, LOD, contamination, high BMI with uncontrolled comorbidities
- Concomitant strategy (same sitting). Simultaneous bariatric and hernia surgery is safe in selected patients with small, uncomplicated hernias.
  - Rationale: avoids second anesthesia and adhesiolysis; useful for small, uncomplicated primary/port-site hernias not requiring wide dissection.
  - Caveats: mesh contamination risk in gastric bypass; technical crowding; higher SSO risk if defects are large.
- Hernia-first strategy.
  - Rarely indicated except for acute incarceration/strangulation or highly symptomatic large LOD precluding safe bariatric access.

13.7.1 Evidence Summary

Population-level and institutional series consistently show worse outcomes when ventral hernia repair precedes bariatric surgery in patients who are otherwise candidates for weight loss surgery. Concomitant repair is feasible and safe for small, simple hernias in expert hands; complex or contaminated reconstructions are better staged. After significant weight loss (typically 9–18 months), reconstructive planes become accessible; wound morbidity falls, and durable meshes can be placed extraperitoneally with lower recurrence [1, 14–17].

13.8 Operative Approach in Obese and Bariatric Patients

13.8.1 Minimally Invasive Bariatric Surgery as First Step in Staged Strategy

Laparoscopy is the approach of choice of bariatric surgery in obese patients with ventral hernias. The presence of a complex hernia can influence the choice of a bariatric procedure and can make it extremely difficult: sometimes, it is necessary to change the patient's position, the trocars, and the use of instruments or perform the procedure through the hernia sac (Fig. 13.2) [11, 14–18]. When selecting among the various procedures (gastric bypass, sleeve gastrectomy, biliopancreatic diversion, etc.), gastric bypass is preferred for its metabolic efficacy, although sleeve gastrectomy may be easier in the presence of large central hernias.

13.8.2 Open Bariatric Surgery as First Step in Staged Strategy

The open approach, although replaced by the laparoscopic technique in most centers, remains fundamental in selected cases, especially when the abdominal anatomy is significantly altered or the complexity of the hernia requires it.

Open surgery allows greater exposure and control of abdominal structures, enabling a safer and more versatile bariatric procedure in complex hernias.

During open surgery, particular attention must be paid to:

- Minimizing tissue trauma to reduce the risk of infection and seroma.
- Careful management of adhesions to avoid visceral injury.
- Hemostatic control and protection of vital structures.

In a staged procedure—depending on the size and characteristics of the hernia, the patient's general condition, infectious risk, and the expected duration of the operation—the hernia may not be treated immediately. In such cases, the viscera can be protected by direct closure of the sac and skin.

Otherwise, the hernia can be repaired with:

- Direct closure of defects, **if** normal intra-abdominal pressure is **maintained**. Intra-abdominal hypertension, which can lead to abdominal compartment syndrome, may result in catastrophic consequences for the patient.
- Use of intraperitoneal onlay mesh (IPOM) with synthetic, resorbable mesh to bridge the defect and covered by the hernia sac, which can help avoid intra-abdominal hypertension (Fig. 13.3).
- Use of component separation techniques reinforced by permanent synthetic mesh **must be avoided.**

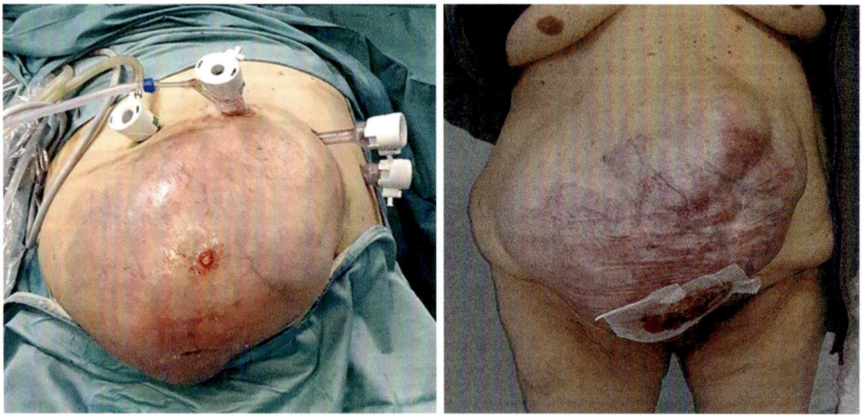

Fig. 13.2 Laparoscopic sleeve gastrectomy trocar position in Class II obese patient with multiple recurrent hernias and loss of domain (LOD)

13.8.3 Open Ventral Hernia Repair

Open repair retains a role for very large defects, hostile abdomens, prior mesh infection, enterocutaneous fistula, or when complex component separation is necessary. Measures to reduce morbidity include:

- Panniculectomy by indication (not routine), meticulous dead-space control, and negative-pressure incision therapy in high-risk wounds [19, 20].
- Anatomical plane selection: retrorectus (sublay) mesh yields better biomechanics and lower recurrence than onlay; consider posterior component separation (transversus abdominis release, TAR) for medialization without extensive skin flaps.
- Drains and quilting sutures to limit seroma [21–23].

13.8.4 Laparoscopic Ventral Hernia Repair (LVHR)

Advantages in obesity include less wound surface, lower infection rates, and faster convalescence [1, 8, 14, 15, 17, 18]. Key technical notes:

- <u>Access</u>: Optical trocar at Palmer's point or left upper quadrant; consider Veress only if adhesiolysis risk is low.
- <u>Adhesiolysis</u>: Sharp, close to parietals; liberal use of energy cautioned in thick fat.
- <u>Defect management</u>: Primary fascial closure (IPOM-plus) when feasible reduces bulge/seroma; otherwise, bridged IPOM with generous overlap (≥5 cm).
- <u>Mesh</u>: Composite barrier meshes for intraperitoneal placement; secure with a measured combination of transfascial sutures and tacks.

Evidence indicates BMI alone should not preclude laparoscopy; outcomes remain favorable across BMI strata when performed by experienced teams.

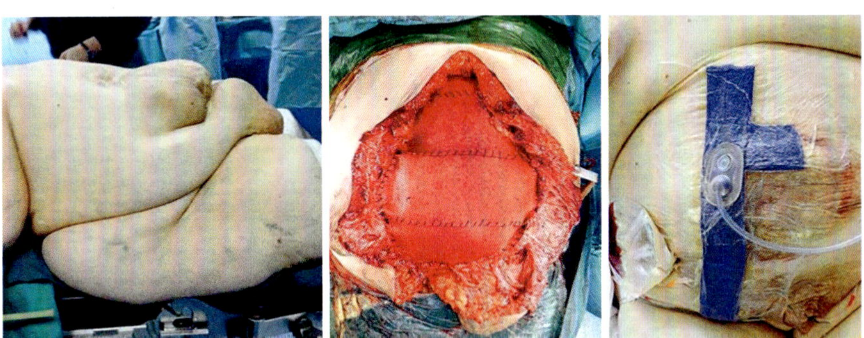

Fig. 13.3 Intraperitoneal onlay mesh (IPOM) repair of complex hernia with polyglycolide-trimethylene carbonate (PGA:TMC) mesh synchronous to open Roux-en-Y gastric bypass

13.8.5 Robotic Ventral Hernia Repair (RVHR)

Robotics expands extraperitoneal options (e.g., r-TAR, robotic extended-view totally extraperitoneal [r-eTEP] ventral, retromuscular/preperitoneal sublay) in obese patients with:

- Enhanced suturing and dissection in thick abdominal walls.
- Low conversion rates and short length of stay even in class III obesity.
- Mesh in the "right" plane (retrorectus/preperitoneal) while maintaining minimally invasive access.

Mid-term series report low recurrence and SSO rates in morbidly obese cohorts, with ergonomic benefits for surgeons. Cost-effectiveness improves with case concentration, shorter stays, and reduced complications [24] (Figs. 13.4 and 13.5).

13.8.6 Hybrid and Adjunct Procedures

- Mini-open retromuscular repair with laparoscopic/robotic assistance to reduce skin flaps.
- Progressive preoperative pneumoperitoneum and botulinum toxin A for LOD to facilitate fascial closure.
- Fasciotens® is a medical device used in ventral hernia repair, particularly for complex cases, by applying controlled vertical traction to the abdominal fascia (Fig. 13.6). Its primary role is to facilitate direct fascial closure of large abdominal wall defects that would otherwise be difficult or impossible to close without significant tension and extensive and invasive surgical techniques [25].
- Targeted panniculectomy/dermolipectomy to improve hygiene and visualization in select patients; not a substitute for weight loss.
- Abdominoplasty combined with repair may be considered after stable weight loss and smoking cessation in carefully selected patients.

13.9 Mesh Selection and Plane of Placement

13.9.1 Mesh Category

- Permanent synthetic (polypropylene, expanded polytetrafluoroethylene [ePTFE], polyvinylidene fluoride [PVDF]): Standard for clean fields; best long-term durability.
- Biosynthetic/long-term absorbable: Option when contamination risk is present and permanent mesh is contraindicated; recurrence higher than permanent synthetics.

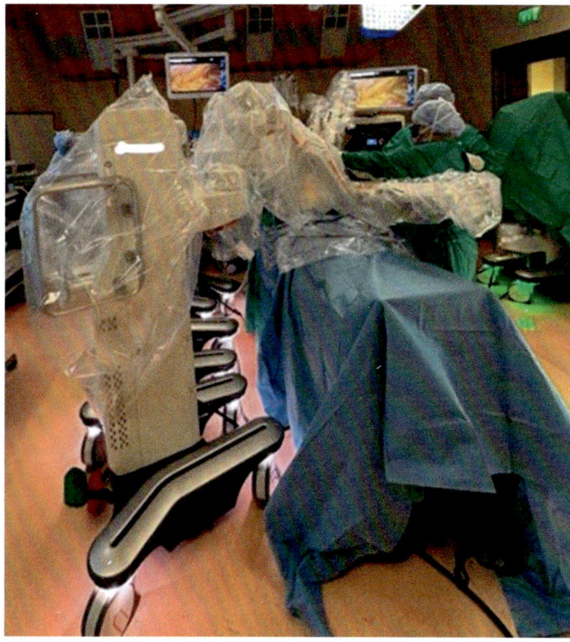

Fig. 13.4 Hugo® Robotic-Assisted Surgery (RAS) system setting in ventral hernia repair

- Biologic: For contamination or bridging when no other option; highest cost and recurrence [26].

13.9.2 Plane

- Retromuscular (sublay): Biomechanically favorable, lower infection/recurrence; achievable open or robotically.
- Preperitoneal: Similar benefits with less posterior sheath dissection; ideal for small-to-moderate defects via robotic cTEP.
- Intraperitoneal (IPOM/IPOM-plus): Useful when extraperitoneal planes are hostile; barrier mesh to minimize adhesions [27].

13.9.3 Fixation

- Extraperitoneal meshes can be sutured or stapled to the posterior sheath with broad overlap.
- Intraperitoneal meshes combine transfascial sutures with limited tacks; excessive tacking can increase pain without improving durability.
- Fascial closure whenever feasible reduces bulge and seroma and improves core function.

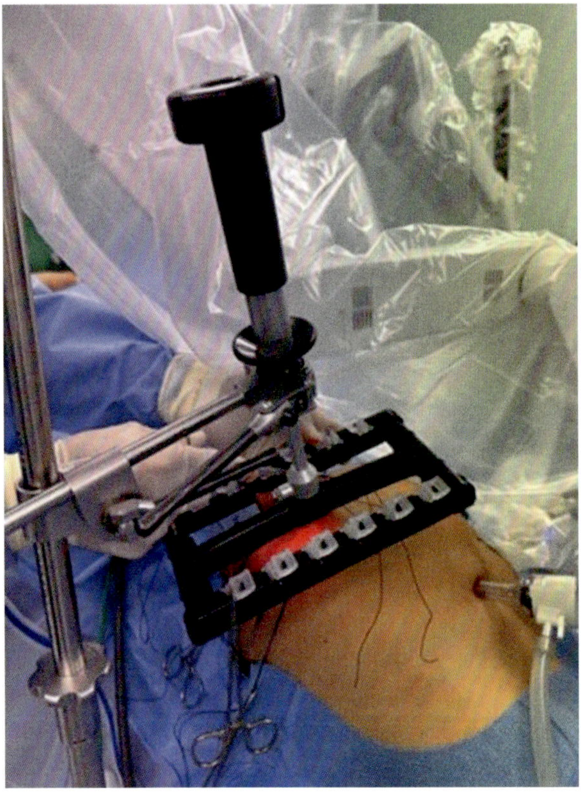

Fig. 13.5 Ventral hernia repair with Xi Da Vinci System® and Fasciotens®

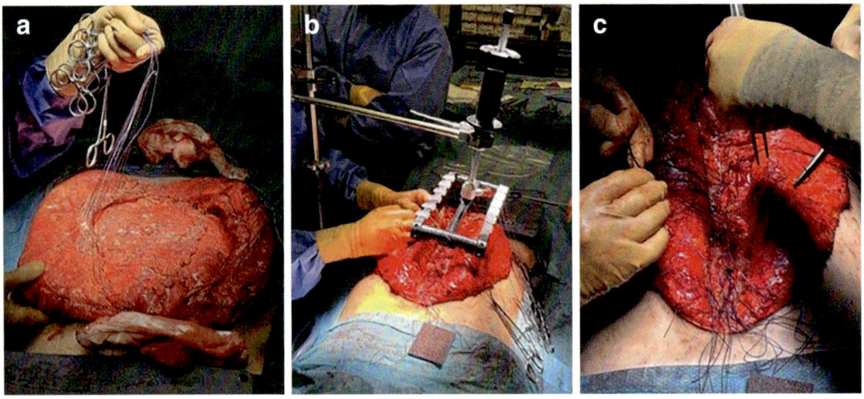

Fig. 13.6 Fasciotens® + transversus abdominis release (TAR) midline closure of a 25 cm W3 hernia defect. (**a**) Sutures are placed on the fascial margins of the hernia defect and connected to the device. (**b**) The device then applies a quantifiable, controlled vertical-diagonal traction to the abdominal wall. (c) This continuous, gentle pull stretches the abdominal wall, elongating the myofascial tissues and counteracting the retraction of the muscle

13.10 Perioperative Anesthesia and ERAS® in Obesity

- Airway & positioning: Ramped intubation, reverse Trendelenburg improves ventilation; utilize longer trocars and thoughtful port geometry in thick abdominal walls.
- Ventilation: Lung-protective strategies (low tidal volumes, PEEP titration), recruitment maneuvers, and postoperative CPAP in OSA.
- Analgesia: Multimodal regimens (acetaminophen, NSAIDs if renal function allows, gabapentinoids selectively); transversus abdominis plane (TAP) blocks or rectus sheath blocks lower opioids and nausea.
- Glycemic management: Basal-bolus insulin protocols and early carbohydrate reintroduction per ERAS®.
- VTE prophylaxis: Higher dose LMW heparin when indicated; consider anti-embolism devices plus early ambulation; extended prophylaxis in very high risk.
- Nausea control and early diet: Aggressive anti-emetic prophylaxis; early liquids/solids as tolerated to accelerate recovery [28, 29].

13.11 Complications, Surveillance, and Mitigation

Surgical-site occurrences (SSOs). Seroma, hematoma, superficial/deep surgical site infection (SSI), and wound dehiscence are more common in high BMI. Prevention: meticulous hemostasis, dead-space control, prophylactic negative-pressure therapy for high-risk incisions, and avoidance of excessive electrocautery in subcutaneous fat.

Chronic pain and bulge. More frequent with bridged IPOM and dense tacking. Strategies: primary closure (IPOM-plus), extraperitoneal mesh planes, and selective neurectomy only after thorough evaluation.

Recurrence. Driven by persistent obesity, large defects, bridged repairs, contaminated fields, and poor glycemic control. Ensure adequate overlap (≥5–7 cm), robust fixation, and—where possible—sublay placement.

Mesh infection. Risk rises with open onlay positions and contamination. Early, aggressive source control; salvage sometimes possible with retromuscular meshes using debridement and negative pressure; explantation when uncontrolled.

Cardiopulmonary/VTE events. Anticipate and prophylaxis: OSA management, early mobilization, appropriate anticoagulation, and hydration.

Post-bariatric considerations. Watch for micronutrient-related delayed healing, anastomotic ulcers (if bypass) influencing NSAID use, and altered drug absorption.

Follow-up. Clinical assessment at 2–4 weeks, 3–6 months, then annually for complex repairs; imaging (US/CT) when symptoms or exam are equivocal. Encourage long-term weight management support.

13.12 Practical Operative Algorithms

Elective ventral/incisional hernia in BMI ≥35 kg/m^2:

1. Optimize (weight loss plan ± bariatric referral, diabetes, smoking cessation, nutrition, OSA).
2. If defect large/complex or contamination risk → stage: bariatric first (if appropriate), defer repair 9–18 months once weight stabilizes.
3. If small, reducible, minimally symptomatic → consider deferring until after weight loss; if symptomatic and patient declines staging, offer minimally invasive repair with full counseling.
4. Preferred planes: retromuscular/preperitoneal (robotic/open as anatomy dictates). If extraperitoneal hostile → IPOM-plus with composite mesh.
5. ERAS® pathway, VTE prophylaxis, postop CPAP where indicated, structured follow-up.

Concomitant bariatric + hernia:

- Limit to small primary or port-site defects; avoid large/complex incisional hernias requiring extensive dissection.
- Use synthetic mesh with extreme caution in contaminated fields; some centers favor primary suture for tiny defects with plan to readdress after weight loss if recurrence occurs.

13.13 Outcomes and Quality Improvement

When BMI is reduced and comorbidities controlled, recurrence rates fall and SSOs decline across approaches. Laparoscopic and robotic repairs consistently shorten length of stay and decrease wound complications compared with open techniques in high-BMI cohorts, while extraperitoneal mesh planes reduce bulge and chronic pain. Multidisciplinary programs (hernia + bariatric + anesthesia + nutrition) and participation in registries/quality collaboratives (where available) enable benchmarking, protocol refinement, and research.

13.14 Future Directions

- Refined risk models incorporating central adiposity metrics, sarcopenic obesity, and glycemic variability to predict SSOs/recurrence.
- Robotic value analyses comparing retromuscular vs IPOM in obesity, with patient-reported outcomes and cost.

- Biomaterials that resist infection and promote integration in compromised soft tissue.
- Prospective trials of staged versus concomitant strategies stratified by hernia size, contamination, and bariatric procedure type.
- Digital prehabilitation (remote nutrition/new drugs/OSA/physical therapy) to scale optimization.

13.15 Conclusion

Abdominal wall surgery in obese and bariatric patients is among the most challenging domains of complex hernia surgery. Evidence consistently highlights the importance of timing (favoring staged repair after weight loss when feasible), optimization of comorbidities, and the use of minimally invasive or robotic techniques. While concomitant repair is feasible in selected cases, careful patient selection is paramount. Future advances will likely be driven by robotic platforms, improved biomaterials, new drugs and instruments, and large-scale outcome data.

References

1. Moszkowicz D, Jacota M, Nkam L, et al. Ventral hernia repair and obesity: results from a nationwide register study in France according to the timeframes of hernia repair and bariatric surgery. Obes Surg. 2021;31(12):5251–9.
2. Brown J, Cornejo J, Zevallos A, et al. Concurrent minimally invasive bariatric surgery and ventral hernia repair with mesh; is it safe? Propensity score matching analysis using the 2015-2022 MBSAQIP database. Surg Endosc. 2024;38(12):7544–51.
3. Parker SG, Mallett S, Quinn L, et al. Identifying predictor of ventral hernia recurrence: systematic review and meta-analysis. BJS Open. 2021;5(2):zraa071.
4. Pernar LI, Pernar CH, Dieffembach BV, et al. What is the BMI threshold for open ventral hernia repair? Surg Endosc. 2017;31(3):1311–7.
5. Haskins IN. Hernia formation: risk factors and biology. Surg Clin North Am. 2023;103(5):835–46.
6. Soare AS, Preda SD, Râmboiu S, et al. Ventral hernia repair and diabetes mellitus – a prospective, observational and comparative study of outcomes. Curr Health Sci J. 2023;49(2):263–72.
7. Kobylińska M, Antosik K, Decyk A, Kurowska K. Malnutrition in obesity: is it possible? Obes Facts. 2022;15(1):19–25.
8. Liang MK, Holihan JL, Itani K, et al. Ventral hernia management: expert consensus guided by systematic review. Ann Surg. 2017;265(1):80–9.
9. Mirghani H, Alamrani SAS, Alkonani AA, Al Madshush AM. The impact of bariatric surgery on weight loss and glycemic control in patients with obesity and type 2 diabetes: a systematic review. Cureus. 2023;15(11):e49122.
10. Alzahrani AAS, Alsoliman MAS, Alattiah TMA, Almohussein NSN. Glycemic control in the era of bariatric surgery: a systematic review and meta-analysis of published studies on the Saudi Arabian population. J Family Med Prim Care. 2024;13(1):15–9.

11. Ghanem OM, Husain F, Chen JY, Lim RB, Kroh M, editors. The SAGES manual of metabolic and bariatric surgery. 3rd ed. Cham: Springer; 2024.
12. Spurzem GJ, Broderick RC, Ruiz-Cota P, et al. GLP-1 receptor agonists are a transformative prehabilitation tool for weight loss in obese patients undergoing elective hernia repair. Surg Endosc. 2025;39(1):440–7.
13. Spurzem GJ, Broderick RC, Ruiz-Cota P, et al. The new bridge to hernia surgery: achieving preoperative weight optimization with GLP-1 receptor agonists for abdominal wall hernia repair. Surg Endosc. 2025;39(8):5296–302.
14. Lomanto D, Shabbir A. Ventral hernia repair in bariatric patients. Minerva Surg. 2021;76(1):17–23.
15. Krivan MS, Giorga A, Barreca M, et al. Concomitant ventral hernia repair and bariatric surgery: a retrospective analysis from a UK-based bariatric center. Surg Endosc. 2019;33(3):705–10.
16. Veilleux E, Lutfi R. Obesity and ventral hernia repair: is there success in staging? J Laparoendosc Adv Surg Tech A. 2020;30(8):896–9.
17. Lazzati A, Nassif GB, Paolino L. Concomitant ventral hernia repair and bariatric surgery: a systematic review. Obes Surg. 2018;28(9):2949–55.
18. Maspero M, Bertoglio CL, Morini L, et al. Laparoscopic ventral hernia repair in patients with obesity: should we be scared of BMI? Surg Endosc. 2022;36(3):2032–41.
19. Xu Y, Shao S, Gong Z, et al. Efficacy of prophylactic negative pressure wound therapy after open ventral hernia repair: a systematic review meta-analysis. BMC Surg. 2023;23(1):374.
20. Mavros MN, Athanasiou S, Alexiou VG, et al. Risk factors for mesh-related infections after hernia repair surgery: a meta-analysis of cohort studies. World J Surg. 2011;35(11):2389–98.
21. Novitsky YW, Elliott HL, Orenstein SB, Rosen MJ. Transversus abdominis muscle release: a novel approach to posterior component separation during complex abdominal wall reconstruction. Am J Surg. 2012;204(5):709–16.
22. Rosen MJ, Denoto G, Itani KM, et al. Evaluation of surgical outcomes of retro-rectus versus intraperitoneal reinforcement with bio-prosthetic mesh in the repair of contaminated ventral hernias. Hernia. 2013;17(1):31–5.
23. Belyansky I, Zahiri HR, Park A. Laparoscopic transversus abdominis release, a novel minimally invasive approach to complex abdominal wall reconstruction. Surg Innov. 2016;23(2):134–41.
24. Gokcal F, Morrison S, Kudsi OY. Robotic ventral hernia repair in morbidly obese patients: perioperative and mid-term outcomes. Surg Endosc. 2020;34(8):3540–9.
25. Niebuhr H, Aufenberg T, Dag H, et al. Intraoperative fascia tension as an alternative to component separation. A prospective observational study. Front Surg. 2021;7:616669.
26. Eriksen JR, Gögenur I, Rosenberg J. Choice of mesh for laparoscopic ventral hernia repair. Hernia. 2007;11(6):481–92.
27. Holihan JL, Nguyen DH, Nguyen MT, et al. Mesh location in open ventral hernia repair: a systematic review and network meta-analysis. World J Surg. 2016;40(1):89–99.
28. Remulla D, Bradley JF 3rd, Henderson W, et al. Consensus in ERAS protocols for ventral hernia repair: evidence-based recommendations from the ACHQC QI Committee. Hernia. 2024;29(1):4.
29. Marcolin P, Mazzola Poli de Figueiredo S, Walmir de Araújo S, et al. Preoperative optimization before ventral hernia repair: a systematic review and meta-analysis. Surg Laparosc Endosc Percutan Tech. 2023;33(2):211–8.

Part IV

Innovative Technologies and Future Perspectives

Tissue Engineering and Regenerative Medicine in Abdominal Wall Reconstruction

14

Corrado Rispoli, Maddalena Claudia Donnarumma, and Nadav Nevo

14.1 Introduction

Complex abdominal wall reconstruction represents not only a technical challenge but also a battle against biology itself. Surgeons routinely encounter hostile soft-tissue environments: open wounds, surgical site infections (SSI), skin necrosis, and high-tension closures. While traditional salvage techniques can control most of the damage, they rarely restore the tissue's full healing potential. Regenerative medicine offers a new opportunity: instead of merely patching or closing abdominal wall defects, we aim to "awaken" the body's own repair mechanisms, leveraging the three pillars of tissue engineering: cells, extracellular matrix and signaling molecules.

Regenerative medicine is an emerging interdisciplinary approach to repairing or replacing damaged or diseased tissues and organs, and it is now spreading widely in all fields of medicine.

Conventional closure methods often fail in contaminated or poorly vascularized fields. Regenerative strategies can transform biologically compromised tissue into an environment primed for orderly healing, thus providing a major contribution in these difficult clinical scenarios.

Total U.S.A. healthcare spending reached approximately $4.9 trillion in 2023, emphasizing the massive economic burden of complex medical care. Chronic wounds alone are estimated to cost $22.5 billion annually, even before accounting for additional expenses related to organ failure or complex reconstructive

C. Rispoli (✉)
Unit of General, Laparoscopic and Robotic Surgery, A.O.R.N. dei Colli Monaldi Hospital, Naples, Italy
e-mail: dott.rispoli@gmail.com

M. C. Donnarumma
General, Mininvasive and Obesity Surgery Unit, University of Campania Luigi Vanvitelli, Naples, Italy

N. Nevo
Department of General Surgery, Sheba Medical Center, Tel Aviv University, Tel Aviv, Israel

D. Cuccurullo, C. Rispoli (eds.), *Complex Abdominal Wall Surgery*, Updates in Surgery, https://doi.org/10.1007/978-3-032-24284-6_14

procedures. This magnitude underscores the urgent need for regenerative solutions capable of improving outcomes and reducing long-term costs [1].

14.2 History and Development of Tissue Engineering and Regenerative Medicine

Regenerative medicine emerged in the first half of the twentieth century, when it was demonstrated that cells, when placed within specific tissue-derived matrices, could survive in heterologous hosts and even partially restore lost physiological functions. A notable example includes pancreatic cells transplanted into a semipermeable envelope for the regulation of glycemia in animal models [2].

In the 1970s and 1980s, the field advanced with the development of the first artificial two-dimensional collagen-based sheets, which could be used to replace damaged skin or other tissues. More recently, technological progress has enabled the fabrication of three-dimensional tissue scaffolds, allowing for more complex and biomimetic regenerative constructs. In recent years, several tissue-engineered skins have received FDA approval, and many other tissues are in advanced stages of clinical trials.

Biological prostheses, such as biological meshes or bioprosthetic materials, have been used in hernia repairs, particularly for complex or contaminated abdominal hernia repairs. They may cause less inflammation and fibrosis compared to synthetic meshes, making them suitable for infected or potentially infected fields [3]. These biological prostheses are typically derived from human (allogenic) or animal (xenogeneic) tissues—such as porcine or bovine—and are processed to remove cellular components, leaving behind a collagen scaffold [4]. However, their main disadvantages are the cost and the relatively high rates of recurrence and complications [5].

14.3 The Biological Rationale: Cells, Matrix, and Signals

When wound healing fails, it is usually because one or more essential ingredients are missing. These can be broadly divided into three categories, according to the specific biological elements they are intended to replace or restore (Fig. 14.1). Effective tissue regeneration requires a coordinated interplay between autologous progenitor cells (such as mesenchymal stem/stromal cells, or MSCs), a supportive matrix, and a proper concentration of growth factors (including platelet-derived growth factor [PDGF], transforming growth factor-beta [TGF-β], and vascular endothelial growth factor [VEGF]).

Each of these elements fuels a positive feedback loop—resolving inflammation, promoting angiogenesis, and guiding collagen maturation. A comprehensive discussion of tissue healing, including its physiological mechanisms and pathological deviations, lies beyond the scope of this chapter. For a more detailed overview, the reader is referred to general textbooks dedicated to the biology of tissue repair.

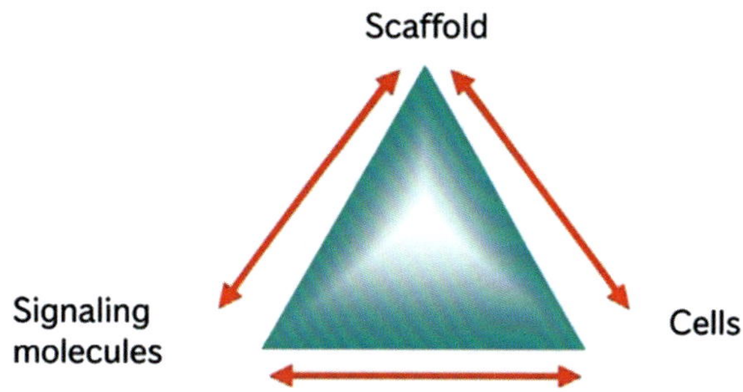

Fig. 14.1 Triad of tissue engineering

Table 14.1 Main origin of stem cells and their characteristics

Origin of steam cells	PROs and CONs
Human embryonic and fetal cells	Few studies; ethical concern
Autologous bone marrow stem cells	Autologous; requires invasive harvesting
Stromal vascular fraction of adipose tissue	Most published; easy harvest; low stem cell proportion (<5%)
Induced pluripotent stem cells	No evidence of *in vivo* use in abdominal wall repair
Adipose-derived mesenchymal stem cell culture	Requires culture; fewer publications than stromal vascular fraction

14.4 Cell-Based Therapies

For over two decades, cell-based therapies have boosted the hopes and aspirations of researchers and healthcare professionals in the field of regenerative medicine. The necessity to develop new treatment options for challenging cases in hernia surgery has created new tools for complex abdominal wall repair (AWR) [6, 7].

Table 14.1 summarizes the main sources of stem cells reported in the literature, with a particular focus on abdominal wall repair.

Each stem cell source presents distinct advantages and limitations, which currently influence their application in clinical AWR.

While clinical evidence remains limited, ongoing trials and translational research are steadily defining the role of cell-based approaches as adjuncts in complex abdominal wall reconstruction, aiming not only to repair the defect but to restore the biological environment necessary for long-term healing.

14.4.1 Adipose-Derived Stromal Vascular Fraction or Mesenchymal Stem Cells

Adipose-derived mesenchymal stem cells (AD-MSCs) are a type of adult stem cell found within adipose tissue. These multipotent cells can differentiate into various mesodermal lineages—such as adipocytes, chondrocytes, osteoblasts, and myocytes—and have shown remarkable potential in promoting angiogenesis, modulating inflammation, and enhancing extracellular matrix remodeling.

AD-MSCs can be isolated from adipose tissue using two principal approaches: enzymatic digestion and mechanical (non-enzymatic) methods. Enzymatic digestion typically employs enzymes such as collagenase or trypsin. The process generally involves washing and mincing the adipose tissue, incubating it with the enzyme at 37 °C, followed by centrifugation and washing steps to isolate the stromal vascular fraction (SVF), from which AD-MSCs are subsequently expanded [8–10]. Mechanical methods avoid proteolytic enzymes and instead rely on approaches such as centrifugation, filtration, micro-fragmentation, or physical emulsification techniques (e.g., Nanofat™, Lipogems™, syringe-based dissociation). These methods vary widely in efficiency, cost, and processing time [11], but have gained widespread use in clinical settings. Enzymatic digestion typically yields a higher number of viable mesenchymal progenitor cells compared to mechanical methods. However, mechanical approaches are considerably faster and potentially more cost-effective, as enzymatic protocols can take up to 210 min and require substantial amounts of reagents. In clinical practice, enzymatic methods are primarily employed in conjunction with cell culture techniques [12]. The cell pellet obtained contains a heterogenous mesodermal cell population consisting of both adipose and hematopoietic stem cells and progenitor cells, as well as other cell types. Preclinical studies demonstrate that these cells enhance angiogenesis and improve collagen quality. Few studies focused on the preclinical (non-human) effect of AD-MSCs in various fields of AWR: notably, some research has focused on their application in mesh integration, where they are seeded onto absorbable or non-absorbable scaffolds to enhance cytocompatibility and tissue regeneration [13, 14]. Probably the main field of application of AD-MSCs is in soft tissue; they have also been injected between dermal tissue and subcutaneous tissue to reduce soft tissue complications [15]. Thanks to their abundance, relative ease of harvest, and low immunogenicity, AD-MSCs have become one of the most studied and clinically promising sources of regenerative cells in the context of AWR and soft tissue reconstruction.

14.4.2 Autologous Micrografts

Autologous micrografts represent an emerging regenerative strategy based on the mechanical disaggregation of small tissue biopsies into viable cellular micro-clusters that retain the capacity to promote tissue repair. These micrografts typically contain keratinocytes, fibroblasts, pericytes, and other stromal cells, maintaining high cell viability (>90%) and preserving the extracellular matrix niche necessary for cellular function and signaling.

Mechanical fragmentation devices, such as MediGraft™ and Rigeneracons™ [16], can process small skin biopsies into micro-fragments (≤80 μm) rich in viable regenerative cell populations [17]. In various fields, such as chronic wound healing, uncontrolled trials showed that the application of micrografts accelerated complete re-epithelialization achieving a notably 75% of complete healing [18]; this evidence can be easily transferred to soft tissue failure during AWR. There are no papers specifically addressing these techniques in AWR, but new experimental studies are ongoing, evaluating micrografts with or without biological and synthetic meshes in small animal models.

14.5 Growth Factor Concentrates

14.5.1 Platelet-Rich Plasma

Platelet-rich plasma (PRP) is a growth factor-rich autologous blood product known to enhance tissue repair through cellular proliferation and neovascularization. It is mainly produced from patient's own blood via centrifugation. PRP harnesses the body's own growth factors to accelerate healing. In animal models, the use of PRP in AWR has been associated with enhanced angiogenesis, myofibroblast recruitment and tissue ingrowth, acellular dermal matrix preservation, less severe peritoneal adhesions, and diminished hernia recurrence. Notably, there is evidence of a reduction in recurrence from 70% to 0% when used in combination with mesh compared to mesh alone [19]. However, there are only a few human studies available with small numbers, or even simple case reports which demonstrate a positive effect of PRP on recurrence of AWR [20]; the available data remain insufficient to draw statistically significant conclusions [21]. More information is available regarding PRP and wound healing, often in complex and chronic scenarios. A meta-analysis of 19 clinical trials found that PRP reduces surgical site infection rates by 32% and halves the time to epithelial closure in clean-contaminated wounds. However, variability in preparation methods remains a challenge [22]. To date, PRP represents the most promising approach for delivering growth factor concentrates in the field of regenerative medicine applied to AWR.

14.5.2 Concentrated Growth Factors

Concentrated growth factors (CGF) are an autologous preparation, obtained from a venous blood sample. They contain high concentrations of growth factors and white blood cells, and not only enhance tissue healing but also improve the clinical outcomes of various surgical procedures, reducing complications like pain, inflammation and morbidity. Similar to PRP, CGF preparation does not involve the use of animal serum, minimizing the risk of infection and immune rejection [23].

CGF have demonstrated a significant impact on the wound-healing potential of human epidermal cells both *in vitro* and *in vivo*; they significantly promote cell proliferation and increase the expression of VEGF and fibroblast growth factor (FGF) [24].

In chronic wound healing CGF has been used in gel and membrane form. CGF gel may accelerate the regeneration of the soft tissue in the wound, although CGF membrane can facilitate its marginal re-epithelialization: when used together, the two forms may support both deep and superficial tissue regeneration [25]. Their role is primary in helping soft tissue failure in AWR (Fig. 14.2).

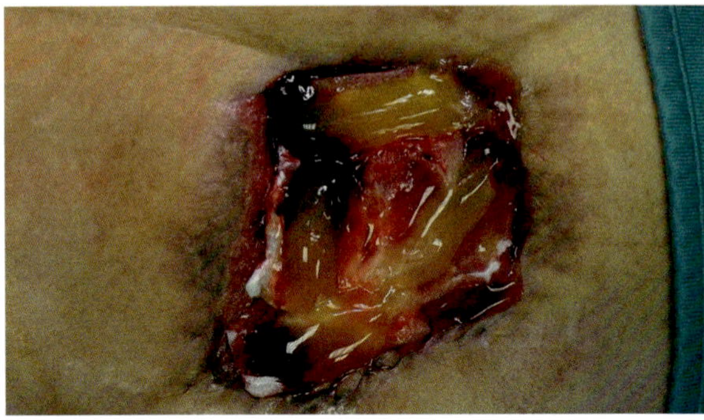

Fig. 14.2 Application of a concentrated growth factor (CGF) gel to accelerate wound healing after infected mesh removal

14.6 Biomaterial Scaffolds

14.6.1 Acellular Dermal Matrices

Acellular dermal matrices (ADMs) are natural tissues that have undergone decellularization to leave behind collagen and extracellular matrix components. ADMs are like a scaffold network that provides support and acts as a framework for the patient's tissues to grow into.

They are mainly derived from animal dermis, through removal of cellular components and tissue engineering strategies aiming at generating dermal tissue resistant to degradation (cross-linking process). A wide range of ADMs are commercially available, derived from heterogeneous dermal sources and subjected to distinct decellularization and processing protocols. Variability in tissue origin and manufacturing methods has been shown to significantly influence the biochemical composition, ultrastructural integrity, and host biological response to the implanted scaffold [26, 27]. Several papers on ADMs in AWR reveal a high heterogeneity of results, but worldwide the main use is in contaminated or infected fields. In some long-term series of more than 700 abdominal wall reconstructions with long-term follow-up, porcine and bovine ADMs provided a 16–20% cumulative hernia recurrence rate—even in highly contaminated (Centers for Disease Control [CDC] III-IV) settings but their use leads to a significant surgical site infection and surgical site occurrence (13–23% and 27–54% respectively) [28, 29].

14.6.2 Bioresorbable Synthetic Scaffolds

Bioresorbable synthetic scaffolds used for the AWR are implantable meshes made from polymers like polyglycolic acid-trimethylene carbonate, which degrade over 12–18 months and are gradually absorbed by the body after supporting tissue repair, without leaving a permanent foreign body. Thanks to their unique features—such as tailorable biodegradation rates, high porosity with varied pore structures, a large surface-to-volume ratio, and adaptable mechanical strength—these polymeric scaffolds have gained considerable attention. They provide important benefits including biological functionality, structural flexibility, and tissue compatibility, which are crucial for tissue engineering and various biomedical applications.

Materials such as polyglycolic acid (PGA), polylactic acid (PLA), and poly-4-hydroxybutyrate (P4HB) have shown favorable biocompatibility, controlled degradation rates, and effective tissue integration [30]. Clinical studies suggest that certain resorbable meshes, like Phasix™ (P4HB), may reduce recurrence rates and improve postoperative outcomes in complex hernia cases compared to biological or permanent synthetic options [31]. However, while bioresorbable scaffolds offer clear advantages in selected patient populations, especially in contaminated fields or high-risk patients, their long-term efficacy and cost-effectiveness remain under investigation [32, 33].

14.7 Future Directions

Looking ahead, the next decade is likely to bring transformative innovations. These may include gene-edited MSCs engineered to enhance angiogenesis, extracellular vesicle therapies that deliver targeted regenerative signals without the need for live cells, and 3D-bioprinted scaffolds tailored to patient-specific anatomy and biomechanics. Smart biomaterials, capable of responding to the local microenvironment through the controlled release of antimicrobials or growth factors, may be especially valuable in contaminated or ischemic fields. Composite scaffolds that mimic the layered architecture of the abdominal wall are also under development, aiming to support more physiological tissue integration.

Additionally, advanced imaging tools help to personalize surgical strategies and optimize long-term outcomes.

Overall, the future of AWR lies in the integration of biologically active materials, autologous cells, and precise surgical planning—moving beyond defect closure toward true tissue regeneration.

14.8 Conclusion

The key for AWR lies not in new materials alone, but in a deeper understanding of how to biologically support and guide tissue regeneration. As clinical experience with regenerative tools expands, the focus will shift from isolated applications to integrated strategies that combine scaffolds, cells, and signaling factors in a rational and patient-specific manner. In this evolving landscape, regenerative medicine is not just an adjunct—it is becoming a framework through which we rethink the entire approach to complex reconstruction. Especially in hostile or contaminated fields, where traditional repairs often fail, regenerative principles offer the possibility of not only closing defects but restoring the tissue's capacity to heal. This paradigm shift will define the next phase of innovation in abdominal wall surgery.

References

1. Sen CK. Human wound and its burden: updated 2025 compendium of estimates. Adv Wound Care (New Rochelle). 2025;14(9):429–38.
2. Chick WL, Like AA, Lauris V. Beta cell culture on synthetic capillaries: an artificial endocrine pancreas. Science. 1975;187(4179):847–9.
3. Wang See C, Kim T, Zhu D. Hernia mesh and hernia repair: a review. Eng Regen. 2020;1:19–33.
4. King KS, Albino FP, Bhanot P. Biologic mesh for abdominal wall reconstruction. Chronic Wound Care Manag Res. 2014;1:57–65.
5. FitzGerald JF, Kumar AS. Biologic versus synthetic mesh reinforcement: what are the pros and cons? Clin Colon Rectal Surg. 2014;27(4):140–8.
6. Petter-Puchner AH, Fortelny RH, Gruber-Blum S, et al. The future of stem cell therapy in hernia and abdominal wall repair. Hernia. 2015;19(1):25–31.
7. Kalaba S, Gerhard E, Winder JS, et al. Design strategies and applications of biomaterials and devices for Hernia repair. Bioact Mater. 2016;1(1):2–17.
8. Bourin P, Bunnell BA, Casteilla L, et al. Stromal cells from the adipose tissue-derived stromal vascular fraction and culture expanded adipose tissue-derived stromal/stem cells: a joint statement of the International Federation for Adipose Therapeutics and Science (IFATS) and the International Society for Cellular Therapy (ISCT). Cytotherapy. 2013;15(6):641–8.
9. Aronowitz JA, Ellenhorn JDI. Adipose stromal vascular fraction isolation: a head-to-head comparison of four commercial cell separation systems. Plast Reconstr Surg. 2013;132(5):932e–9e.
10. Astori G, Vignati F, Bardelli S, et al. "In vitro" and multicolor phenotypic characterization of cell subpopulations identified in fresh human adipose tissue stromal vascular fraction and in the derived mesenchymal stem cells. J Transl Med. 2007;5:55.
11. Aronowitz JA, Lockhart RA, Hakakian CS. Mechanical versus enzymatic isolation of stromal vascular fraction cells from adipose tissue. Springerplus. 2015;4:713.
12. Condé-Green A, Kotamarti VS, Sherman LS, et al. Shift toward mechanical isolation of adipose-derived stromal vascular fraction: review of upcoming techniques. Plast Reconstr Surg Glob Open. 2016;4(9):e1017.
13. Guillaume O, Park J, Monforte X, et al. Fabrication of silk mesh with enhanced cytocompatibility: preliminary in vitro investigation toward cell-based therapy for hernia repair. J Mater Sci Mater Med. 2016;27(2):37.
14. Zanolla I, Tiengo E, Zanotti F, et al. Tissue reconstruction of abdominal wall with butyric acid-based nets: preliminary in vitro test using tissue engineering strategies. Eur Rev Med Pharmacol Sci. 2022;26(3 Suppl):11–20.
15. Sheng L, Yang M, Li H, et al. Transplantation of adipose stromal cells promotes neovascularization of random skin flaps. Tohoku J Exp Med. 2011;224(3):229–34.
16. Trovato L, Monti M, Del Fante C, et al. A new medical device rigeneracons allows to obtain viable micro-grafts from mechanical disaggregation of human tissues. J Cell Physiol. 2015;230(10):2299–303.
17. Purpura V, Bondioli E, Graziano A, et al. Tissue characterization after a new disaggregation method for skin micro-grafts generation. J Vis Exp. 2016;(109):e53579.
18. Baglioni EA, Perego F, Paolin E, et al. Efficacy of autologous micrografts technology: a promising approach for chronic wound healing and tissue regeneration-a pilot study. Front Med. 2024;11:1417920.
19. Van Eps J, Fernandez-Moure J, Cabrera F, et al. Decreased hernia recurrence using autologous platelet-rich plasma (PRP) with Strattice™ mesh in a rodent ventral hernia model. Surg Endosc. 2016;30(8):3239–49.
20. Anestiadou E, Kotidis E, Abba Deka I, et al. Platelet-rich therapies in hernia repair: a comprehensive review of the impact of platelet concentrates on mesh integration in hernia management. Biomolecules. 2024;14(8):921.

21. Popescu V, Pătraşcu T, Andraş D, et al. Plasma derived products for polypropylene mesh integration in abdominal wall defects: procedure description and partial results. Chirurgia (Bucur). 2021;116(5):599–608.
22. Azzena B, Mazzoleni F, Abatangelo G, et al. Autologous platelet-rich plasma as an adipocyte in vivo delivery system: case report. Aesth Plast Surg. 2008;32(1):155–8.
23. Xu C, Pei Y, Wang Y, et al. Progress in the application of auto-concentrated growth factor (CGF) in wound repair. J Biomater Appl. 2025;39(8):819–27.
24. Liu Y, Liu Y, Zeng C, Li W, Ke C, Xu S. Concentrated growth factor promotes wound healing potential of HaCaT Cells by activating the RAS signaling pathway. Front Biosci (Landmark Ed). 2022;27(12):319.
25. Kao CH. Use of concentrate growth factors gel or membrane in chronic wound healing: description of 18 cases. Int Wound J. 2020;17(1):158–66.
26. Ott HC, Rajab TK. Tissue-derived matrices. In: Lee SJ, Yoo JJ, Atala A, editors. In situ tissue regeneration. London: Academic; 2016. p. 229–50.
27. Shankaran V, Weber DJ, Reed RL 2nd, Luchette FA. A review of available prosthetics for ventral hernia repair. Ann Surg. 2011;253(1):16–26.
28. Asaad M, Kapur SK, Baumann DP, et al. Acellular dermal matrix provides durable long-term outcomes in abdominal wall reconstruction: a study of patients with over 60 months of follow-up. Ann Surg. 2022;276(5):e563–70.
29. Hassan AM, Asaad M, Seitz AJ, et al. Effect of wound contamination on outcomes of abdominal wall reconstruction using acellular dermal matrix: 14-year experience with more than 700 patients. J Am Coll Surg. 2021;233(6):676–84.
30. Pogson-Morowitz K, Porras Fimbres D, Barrow BE, et al. Contemporary abdominal wall reconstruction: emerging techniques and trends. J Clin Med. 2024;13(10):2876.
31. Roth JS, Anthone GJ, Selzer DJ, et al. Prospective, multicenter study of P4HB (Phasix™) mesh for hernia repair in cohort at risk for complications: 3-year follow-up. Ann Med Surg (Lond). 2020;61:1–7.
32. Saiding Q, Chen Y, Wang J, et al. Abdominal wall hernia repair: from prosthetic meshes to smart materials. Mater Today Bio. 2023;21:100691.
33. Serrano-Aroca Á, Pous-Serrano S. Prosthetic meshes for hernia repair: state of art, classification, biomaterials, antimicrobial approaches, and fabrication methods. J Biomed Mater Res A. 2021;109(12):2695–719.

Enhanced Recovery After Surgery (ERAS®) in Abdominal Wall Reconstruction: Evidence-Based Clinical Guidelines

15

Nadav Nevo and Corrado Rispoli

15.1 Introduction

Abdominal wall reconstruction (AWR) frequently involves patients with multiple comorbidities and large, complex hernias—features associated with higher wound morbidity and prolonged hospitalization. Enhanced Recovery After Surgery (ERAS®) pathways standardize perioperative care, attenuate the surgical stress response, and improve recovery time. In ventral hernia/AWR populations, ERAS® implementation has been associated with shorter length of stay (LOS) and fewer complications, without higher readmissions, and with meaningful potential for cost containment given the substantial economic burden of incisional hernia care [1–4].

This chapter is structured with a practical approach, similar to a guideline, and includes real-life protocols. For each key point, a brief description is provided and a recommendation is given to support the adoption of the ERAS® approach

15.2 Preoperative Optimization

15.2.1 Nutritional Optimization

Malnutrition is a recognized risk factor for postoperative complications, particularly in patients undergoing major abdominal surgery and AWR. Deficits in protein and energy balance impair wound healing, increase susceptibility to infections, and prolong hospitalization. Hypoalbuminemia, a common surrogate marker for poor

N. Nevo (✉)
Department of General Surgery, Sheba Medical Center, Tel Aviv University, Tel Aviv, Israel
e-mail: nadav.nevo@sheba.health.gov.il

C. Rispoli
Unit of General, Laparoscopic and Robotic Surgery, A.O.R.N. dei Colli Monaldi Hospital, Naples, Italy

D. Cuccurullo, C. Rispoli (eds.), *Complex Abdominal Wall Surgery*, Updates in Surgery, https://doi.org/10.1007/978-3-032-24284-6_15

nutritional status, is strongly correlated with surgical site infections (SSI), prolonged LOS, and worse overall outcomes. In high-risk populations, preoperative nutritional interventions, especially immunonutrition enriched with arginine, omega-3 fatty acids, and nucleotides, have been shown to modulate immune response and reduce infectious morbidity. Evidence indicates that a short course (5–7 days) of perioperative immunonutrition in malnourished patients improves wound healing and reduces SSI. Given the high incidence of malnutrition in complex hernia patients, nutritional optimization represents a critical first step in ERAS® protocols.

15.2.1.1 Key Evidence

- Low preoperative albumin is associated with higher SSI and longer LOS after ventral/incisional hernia repair [5, 6].
- The European Society for Clinical Nutrition and Metabolism (ESPEN) guidelines recommend 5–7 days of enteral immunonutrition for malnourished surgical patients [7].

15.2.1.2 Recommendation

- Defer elective AWR when feasible until nutritional status is optimized (e.g., albumin >3.5 g/dL).
- Provide 5–7 days of preoperative immunonutrition for malnourished patients [7].

15.2.2 Smoking Cessation

Tobacco use is a well-established modifiable risk factor in surgical patients, with serious effects on wound healing and mesh integration. Nicotine-induced vasoconstriction reduces tissue oxygenation, while carbon monoxide lowers oxygen delivery, both impairing fibroblast proliferation and collagen synthesis. Smokers undergoing AWR demonstrate increased rates of wound dehiscence, mesh infections, and hernia recurrence compared with nonsmokers. Multiple studies across surgical populations confirm that cessation for at least 4 weeks significantly reduces postoperative complications, with further benefit observed after 8 weeks. The addition of pharmacologic agents such as varenicline to behavioral support doubles the success rates of smoking cessation compared to counseling alone, although it may lengthen the overall cessation process. Incorporating structured smoking cessation programs into preoperative optimization is therefore a cornerstone of ERAS.

15.2.2.1 Key Evidence

- Smoking increases wound complications and mesh-related morbidity in surgical patients, including hernia cohorts [8, 9].
- ≥4–8 weeks of cessation reduces postoperative risk; pharmacologic + behavioral interventions improve quit rates [10, 11].

15.2.2.2 Recommendation

- Require ≥4 weeks of verified abstinence before elective AWR; ≥8 weeks is ideal.
- Offer combined pharmacologic and behavioral cessation support [10, 11].

15.2.3 Glycemic Control

Glycemic regulation plays a pivotal role in surgical recovery, particularly in operations with a high risk of wound morbidity such as AWR. Hyperglycemia impairs innate immunity by disrupting neutrophil function and increases oxidative stress, both of which contribute to impaired collagen synthesis and defective wound healing. In general surgical cohorts, perioperative glucose levels >180 mg/dL are consistently associated with higher SSI rates, prolonged LOS, and increased risk of sepsis. In addition to perioperative glucose control, longterm glycemic status is equally important: patients with $HbA_{1c} \geq 7\%$ demonstrate significantly higher infectious complication rates than those with optimal control. For patients undergoing complex hernia repair, who often require prosthetic materials, even mild hyperglycemia may predispose to graft infections and wound breakdown. Therefore, ERAS® emphasize s careful yet effective perioperative glucose monitoring and long-term glycemic optimization as dual strategies to improve outcomes.

15.2.3.1 Key Evidence

- Postoperative glucose >180 mg/dL is associated with higher SSI risk in general surgical patients [12].
- $HbA_{1c} \geq 7\%$ correlates with more infectious complications across surgical cohorts [13].

15.2.3.2 Recommendation

- Maintain perioperative glucose <180 mg/dL whenever possible.
- Optimize $HbA_{1c} < 7\%$ before elective AWR [12, 13].

15.3 Intraoperative Management

15.3.1 Minimally Invasive Techniques

Minimally invasive surgery has transformed ventral hernia and abdominal wall reconstruction. Compared with open repair, laparoscopy reduces wound morbidity, lowers SSI rates, and shortens recovery. A landmark randomized VA (Veterans Administration) trial confirmed fewer complications with laparoscopic repair, establishing its role in suitable patients. Robotic-assisted approaches have since broadened the minimally invasive armamentarium, offering enhanced dexterity and ergonomics. Contemporary randomized and prospective studies indicate that robotic and laparoscopic repair achieve comparable short-term outcomes in terms of safety and recurrence, though robotic repair may be associated with longer operative times and higher costs. In complex hernias, however, the robotic platform may facilitate difficult reconstructions. The choice of minimally invasive approach should therefore be tailored to defect characteristics, patient risk profile, and institutional expertise.

15.3.1.1 Key Evidence

- Laparoscopy: lower wound complications compared with open repair [14].
- Robotics vs. laparoscopy: comparable outcomes in RCTs; robotic repair associated with longer operative times and higher costs [15, 16].

15.3.1.2 Recommendation

- Prefer a minimally invasive approach when feasible, tailoring to patient and defect characteristics.

15.3.2 Multimodal Analgesia

Pain control is central to recovery, and ERAS® protocols emphasize opioid-sparing multimodal analgesia. The rationale is twofold: improved pain control enables earlier mobilization, and minimizing opioids reduces ileus, respiratory depression, and dependency risks. Regional techniques, such as transversus abdominis plane (TAP) blocks, significantly reduce opioid consumption and pain scores following abdominal surgery. Adjuvants such as low-dose ketamine have been shown to reduce acute postoperative pain and opioid requirements without major adverse effects. Non-opioid systemic agents, including acetaminophen and NSAIDs, are safe and effective when scheduled, providing a foundation upon which regional and adjunctive techniques can be layered. A balanced analgesic regimen therefore enhances both comfort and functional recovery in AWR.

15.3.2.1 Key Evidence

- TAP blocks: reduced opioid use and pain [17].
- Ketamine: effective analgesic adjunct [18].

15.3.2.2 Recommendation

- Use TAP blocks with scheduled acetaminophen/NSAIDs; consider low-dose ketamine selectively.

15.4 Postoperative Recovery

15.4.1 Early Enteral Nutrition

Early enteral feeding is a hallmark of ERAS®, based on strong evidence that it reduces postoperative ileus, supports gut integrity, and accelerates recovery. Traditionally delayed due to concerns about bowel function, early feeding has now been shown to be both safe and well tolerated after abdominal surgery, including ventral hernia repair. Starting clear liquids on the day of surgery and advancing as tolerated promotes faster return of gastrointestinal function, reduces infection rates, and shortens LOS. For AWR patients, who often undergo large dissections with significant physiological stress, early nutrition helps maintain nitrogen balance and supports wound healing.

15.4.1.1 Recommendation

- Initiate oral/enteral feeding on postoperative day 0, advancing as tolerated within ERAS® protocols [2, 3, 19].

15.4.2 Early Mobilization

Prolonged bed rest is strongly associated with complications such as pneumonia, thromboembolism, and muscle atrophy. ERAS® emphasizes early and structured mobilization to counter these risks. Studies across surgical populations demonstrate that ambulation on the day of surgery, with progressive daily mobility goals, leads to shorter LOS and fewer complications. In AWR, early mobilization not only improves respiratory function but also reduces risks of ileus and thromboembolic events. Clear communication of mobility targets and interdisciplinary support (nursing, physiotherapy) are crucial for adherence.

15.4.2.1 Recommendation

- Encourage ambulation on the day of surgery and establish daily mobility goals [20].

15.4.3 Respiratory Physiotherapy

Pulmonary complications remain a significant contributor to morbidity in patients undergoing major abdominal wall reconstruction, particularly those with obesity, COPD, or extensive open repairs. A systematic review for the American College of Physicians demonstrated that postoperative pulmonary complications (PPCs) are as frequent and clinically important as cardiac complications, and are associated with increased morbidity, mortality, and prolonged hospital stay. Interventions such as incentive spirometry, deep breathing exercises, continuous positive airway pressure therapy, and chest physiotherapy are widely adopted. Evidence for lung-expansion strategies shows some benefit in reducing PPCs, particularly in high-risk patients, though the overall quality of studies is variable and results are not uniformly consistent. Within ERAS® pathways, selective and targeted physiotherapy remains a rational approach given the high prevalence of pulmonary comorbidities in abdominal wall reconstruction.

15.4.3.1 Key Evidence

- PPCs are common after abdominal surgery and significantly increase morbidity, mortality, and hospital length of stay.
- Lung-expansion and physiotherapy interventions may reduce PPCs in high-risk patients, though study results are inconsistent [21].

15.4.3.2 Recommendation

- Consider routine postoperative respiratory physiotherapy in high-risk patients.
- Individualize interventions, recognizing heterogeneity in evidence quality and patient risk profiles.

Summary Box

Phase	Recommendation	Impact/key finding	Supporting references
Preoperative	Optimize nutrition; defer surgery if albumin ≤3.5 g/dL	Low albumin associated with ↑ SSI and ↑ LOS after ventral/incisional hernia repair	[5, 6]
Preoperative	Immunonutrition (arginine, ω-3, nucleotides) for malnourished patients, 5–7 days	Fewer infectious complications in malnourished surgical patients	[7]
Preoperative	Smoking cessation ≥4 weeks (≥8 weeks ideal); pharmacologic + behavioral support	Lower postoperative complications; effective cessation with varenicline/ combined support	[8–11]
Preoperative	Glycemic optimization: HbA_{1c} <7% preoperative; maintain perioperative glucose <180 mg/dL	Lower SSI with better glycemic control	[12, 13]
Intraoperative	Prefer minimally invasive repair (laparoscopic/robotic) when feasible	Lower wound morbidity vs. open; comparable outcomes robotics vs. laparoscopy in RCTs	[14–16]
Intraoperative	Multimodal analgesia with TAP block; scheduled acetaminophen/NSAIDs; ketamine	Reduced pain and opioid consumption; effective adjunct with ketamine	[17, 18]
Postoperative	Early oral/enteral feeding (POD 0), advance as tolerated	Reduced ileus and faster GI recovery; good tolerance in VHR ERAS implementations	[2, 3, 19]
Postoperative	Early mobilization with daily goals	Shorter LOS; fewer complications	[20]
Postoperative	Respiratory physiotherapy in high-risk patients	May reduce pulmonary complications, though evidence is mixed	[21]

ERAS® Enhanced Recovery After Surgery, *GI* gastrointestinal, *LOS* length of stay, *POD* postoperative day, *SSI* surgical site infection, *TAP* transversus abdominis plane, *VHR* ventral hernia repair

References

1. Lode L, Oma E, Henriksen NA, Jensen KK. Enhanced recovery pathways in abdominal wall reconstruction: a systematic review and meta-analysis. Surg Endosc. 2021;35(2):514–23.
2. Majumder A, Fayezizadeh M, Neupane R, et al. Benefits of multimodal enhanced recovery pathway in patients undergoing open ventral hernia repair. J Am Coll Surg. 2016;222(6):1106–15.
3. Stearns E, Plymale MA, Davenport DL, et al. Early outcomes of an enhanced recovery protocol for open repair of ventral hernia. Surg Endosc. 2018;32(6):2914–22.
4. Gillion JF, Sanders D, Miserez M, Muysoms F. The economic burden of incisional ventral hernia repair: a multicenter cost analysis. Hernia. 2016;20(6):819–30.
5. Dunne JR, Malone DL, Tracy JK, et al. Abdominal wall hernias: risk factors for infection and resource utilization. J Surg Res. 2003;111(1):78–84.
6. Kaoutzanis C, Leichtle SW, Mouawad NJ, et al. Risk factors for postoperative wound infections and prolonged hospitalization after ventral/incisional hernia repair. Hernia. 2015;19(1):113–23.
7. Weimann A, Braga M, Carli F, et al. ESPEN guideline: clinical nutrition in surgery. Clin Nutr. 2017;36(3):623–50.
8. Hawn MT, Houston TK, Campagna EJ, et al. The attributable risk of smoking on surgical complications. Ann Surg. 2011;254(6):914–20.
9. Sørensen LT. Wound healing and infection in surgery: the pathophysiological impact of smoking, smoking cessation, and nicotine replacement therapy: a systematic review. Ann Surg. 2012;255(6):1069–79.
10. Thomsen T, Villebro N, Møller AM. Interventions for preoperative smoking cessation. Cochrane Database Syst Rev. 2014;2014(3):CD002294.
11. Cahill K, Stevens S, Perera R, Lancaster T. Pharmacological interventions for smoking cessation: overview and network meta-analysis. Cochrane Database Syst Rev. 2013;2013(5):CD009329.
12. Ata A, Lee J, Bestle SL, et al. Postoperative hyperglycemia and surgical site infection in general surgery patients. Arch Surg. 2010;145(9):858–64.
13. Dronge AS, Perkal MF, Kancir S, et al. Long-term glycemic control and postoperative infectious complications. Arch Surg. 2006;141(4):375–80.
14. Itani KMF, Hur K, Kim LT, et al. Comparison of laparoscopic and open repair with mesh for the treatment of ventral incisional hernia: a randomized trial. Arch Surg. 2010;145(4):322–8
15. Petro CC, Zolin S, Krpata D, et al. Patient-reported outcomes of robotic vs laparoscopic ventral hernia repair with intraperitoneal mesh: the PROVE-IT randomized clinical trial. JAMA Surg. 2021;156(1):22–9.
16. Dhanani NH, Lyons NB, Olavarria OA, et al. Robotic versus laparoscopic ventral hernia repair: two-year results from a prospective, multicenter, blinded randomized clinical trial. Ann Surg. 2023;278(2):161–5.
17. Abdallah FW, Chan VW, Brull R. Transversus abdominis plane block: a systematic review. Reg Anesth Pain Med. 2012;37(2):193–209.
18. Brinck ECV, Tiippana E, Heesen M, et al. Perioperative intravenous ketamine for acute postoperative pain in adults. Cochrane Database Syst Rev. 2018;12(12):CD012033.
19. Lewis SJ, Andersen HK, Thomas S. Early enteral nutrition within 24 h of intestinal surgery versus later commencement of feeding: a systematic review and meta-analysis. J Gastrointest Surg. 2009;13(3):569–75.
20. Hoyer EH, Friedman M, Lavezza A, et al. Promoting mobility and reducing length of stay in hospitalized general medicine patients: a quality-improvement project. J Hosp Med. 2016;11(5):341–7.
21. Lawrence VA, Cornell JE, Smetana GW, American College of Physicians. Strategies to reduce postoperative pulmonary complications after noncardiothoracic surgery: systematic review for the American College of Physicians. Ann Intern Med. 2006;144(8):596–608.

SPRINGER NATURE

GPSR Compliance

The European Union's (EU) General Product Safety Regulation (GPSR) is a set of rules that requires consumer products to be safe and our obligations to ensure this.

If you have any concerns about our products, you can contact us on ProductSafety@springernature.com

In case Publisher is established outside the EU, the EU authorized representative is:

Springer Nature Customer Service Center GmbH
Europaplatz 3
69115 Heidelberg, Germany

Printed by Wilco bv, the Netherlands